THE COMPLETE INSULIN RESISTANCE DIET FOR PCOS

A No-Stress Meal Plan with Easy Recipes to Stop PCOS Symptoms, Repair Your Metabolism, and Lose Weight Naturally

By Maggie Glisson

TABLE OF CONTENTS

INTRODUCTION

Welcome back! I would like to start by saying thank you so much to all of the readers who are here after reading my first book, *The PCOS Fix*. Writing that book transformed my life completely. It connected me to a supportive community and made me look at some of my long-held beliefs about health, happiness, and daily habits. In particular, it revolutionized my relationship with food. Sharing that journey with you has been one of the highlights of my life, and that is why I decided to follow up with another book; this time focused on recipes.

After writing *The PCOS Fix*, I realized there was so much more information on diet, metabolism, and weight I wanted to include. I knew I had to write another book in which I could share practical recipes and methods to support change. This book has been written as a complement to the first book, but is also helpful on its own.

For those who don't know me yet, my name is Maggie Glisson and the reason I was inspired to support women with PCOS is that, until recently, I was in the same position as you probably are now. I had a million questions after my diagnosis, and not very many answers.

My story began just over five years ago. I was in my early thirties, and my partner and I had been trying to get pregnant for around a year. We were not particularly worried at that point. I had only come off the contraceptive pill about 12 months earlier and we were aware that it could take time for my fertility levels to return to normal. So, neither of us was particularly anxious during the initial trip to the doctor. I expected it to be an informal chat about my health and to get the green light to continue our baby-making efforts, safe in the knowledge that time was all that was needed to solve this problem.

Instead, it ended up being an in-depth fact-finding mission that involved uncomfortable questions about my health—areas that I knew had been an issue but in no way thought were related to my chances of getting pregnant. But as he asked question after question, and as I reflected on my general, mental, and physical health, a cold feeling crept over my entire body, to the point that when he finished speaking, I was sure I hadn't heard a word he'd said for the last twenty minutes. It was as if it all finally made sense, and I had known all along that there must be some connection between all these facets of my life.

As a teenager, it felt like my life was governed by two things: my weight and my emotions. With a diet sky-high in sugar and processed food and with years to go before the average person knew about the impact these foods would have, I was completely ignorant about the effects my lifestyle choices were having on my long-term health. My mood swings and tendency to burst into tears at a moment's notice were labeled as a normal part of puberty. This theory was backed up by the fact that so many of my girlfriends seemed to be going through similar experiences. We were assured by parents, teachers, and each other that this was all just part of growing up, and as soon as we were older, our bodies would normalize and our emotions would even out.

Fast forward to my mid-twenties, where my body had normalized for sure. My new normal was an extra 15-25 pounds that I carried mostly around my stomach. It became so normal I stopped noticing. Every few years, I would creep up a dress size. I would jump from one fad diet to another with no results other than an extra few pounds. This was due in part to the fact that I never stuck to one dietary plan for long, and that whenever I tried to cut down on sugary treats or bread, I would be so miserable that I would quickly pick it back up again.

Again, most of my girlfriends had the same issues. This was back in the days when the internet had just cemented itself as a part of our daily routines, and social media was starting to grow popular. So, I could see that not only were some of the women in my family and social circle prone to weight gain but other women as well! This pattern only added to my confidence that there was nothing wrong with me in particular—weight gain, and what seemed like complete immunity to the effects of exercise were just normal parts of being in your twenties. Plus, by that point, I had already met my husband-to-be, and we were happy. So why worry so much about my weight if there was nothing I could do to change it?

The emotional symptoms were a bit harder to explain away. I had progressed out of the teenage phase of bursting into tears at the drop of a hat, but that had been replaced with a slow-growing, ever-present, and sometimes overwhelming feeling of unhappiness and discontent. It grew so steadily during my early twenties that I almost didn't notice it. But by the time I was approaching my thirties, getting married, and considering starting a family, it had taken over so much of my thought process and mental health that I had already reached out to medical professionals for help.

As a woman in her late twenties, I was now refusing to hear that my problems were normal or that I would grow out of them. My thirties were approaching. Surely my time for growing out of things was long behind me! Some of the strategies I tried worked temporarily, some didn't work at all, and others I refused to even try. Again, as with the weight, after a while I assumed that this was just the way I was. And hey, every couple argued, and there were times when I was upset over things that could be considered legitimate concerns. No way could this all be connected to any physical problem. This was just part of life.

Now into my early thirties, imagine my moment of absolute clarity in that doctor's office when my answers to all of his questions around my health were that it was *"Just the way I was."* The weight; the depression; the emotional overreaction; the acne; the debilitating pain during my period; the irregular and sometimes absent periods; the irrational fights with my husband. These things were not just me being me—these were symptoms. These were symptoms of PCOS that I had actually been trying to normalize since I was 13 years old.

Getting a medical diagnosis can feel like you have the proverbial weight taken off your shoulders. But realizing that this diagnosis could now spell infertility was like having that weight, and then some, replaced. Okay, this was my life now. This was us starting the journey of looking at other medical options in order to get pregnant. This was our time to start using the words in vitro fertilization, surrogacy, or even adoption.

Or was it?

Over the years, I had researched natural treatments for my depressive episodes and general mental health. In the process, I had become increasingly aware of holistic approaches for a wide range of female health conditions. I started to think about the information I might find if I looked into possible treatments for PCOS. Was there a chance that maybe, just maybe, I would be able to heal, and possibly even have a family naturally?

That's when I came across Italian fashion influencer Chiara Ferragni's story. She had battled with PCOS, and won: she got pregnant and had a child. Stories like this are now more common, but at the time it sparked my fascination with what can be achieved by making changes in my life.

And so I began my journey into the online world of PCOS information and support. It is a journey that I am still on to this very day, although my reasons for continuing have changed. You see, I've already received my miracle. I have a healthy, happy baby who was conceived naturally and delivered with no complications. For many women, their PCOS journey would have ended there. But for me, it was not just about achieving that goal, although I can't even tell you how much joy and happiness our son has brought in to our lives. For me, it was also about getting my life back: enjoying great health, learning to love myself, and improving my personal relationships. That part of my journey surprised me the most.

That is why I have made it my mission to share my knowledge and experience with other women, like you. That is why I now feel confident and empowered to share my story. If becoming pregnant is your goal, then this book can help with that. But there is more to PCOS than fertility problems, and I want to raise awareness of how recognizing, managing, and overcoming the symptoms of PCOS will radically transform almost every area of your life.

In *The PCOS Fix*, I wrote about how PCOS generally impacts on your life and what you can do about it. Now, I want to delve further into food, while also focusing on practical tips. That's why I have created this compendium cookbook, which comes with a full 30-day PCOS Boot Camp. My aim here is to support you to start using food as a tool for healing. You will find a variety of delicious recipes, as well as preparation, cooking, and sourcing tips. Change can be challenging, and one of the most important factors when you begin switching your diet is to figure out how it can fit into your daily routine. That is why I created the 30-Day PCOS Boot Camp, which will guide you to put changes into practice and start healing your symptoms today.

Whether you are a new reader, or a returning follower, I look forward to taking you through an intensive but fun overhaul of your kitchen and your life!

It was so much fun designing the 30-Day PCOS Boot Camp. I only wish information like this had been available when I was first diagnosed. It is my greatest wish that you find this content helpful, so please make sure you leave a review and let me know what you think.

Right, we're almost ready to dive into it. In the first chapter, we'll look at the effect of insulin on health and weight. I will discuss the lifestyle changes needed to heal PCOS, to give you an overview of what to expect if you choose to go on this journey (I certainly hope you do!). This book is intended as a guide to help you navigate your post-diagnosis world. If you decide to implement the changes discussed in this book, please do so as an ongoing exercise - for change to translate into positive effects, it has to be sustained and long-term. Take action today, and you will free yourself from the grip of PCOS and create the healthy life you want.

Thank you again for making me part of your

journey. I wish you the best of luck with the second stage of your PCOS lifestyle transformation!

Let's get started.

CHAPTER ONE

HOW AND WHY INSULIN RESISTANCE MAKES US FAT

By now, you should have a general idea that insulin resistance is not a good thing. Not only is it harmful to your health, it exacerbates PCOS. But how? This may be something you are not familiar with unless you or a family member has had issues with insulin resistance or diabetes.

While scientists have researched this area extensively, they haven't concluded whether PCOS is caused by insulin resistance, or whether insulin resistance causes PCOS. They are so entwined, it could be argued that the order of cause and effect is not important. Rather, what is important is to be aware of how our own habits increase the chance of insulin resistance… and how we can avoid it.

In this chapter, I will explore insulin resistance in more detail: what it is, how it happens, and why it so often leads to weight gain. From this foundation of knowledge, we'll then create a new diet that will tackle insulin resistance and help you manage your PCOS symptoms.

What is Insulin Resistance?

When you eat food, your digestion breaks it down into smaller molecules that your body can make use of. One of these is glucose. When your pancreas detects elevated levels of glucose in your blood, it produces insulin. Insulin is a hormone that instructs your cells to absorb and make use of that glucose for energy. If there is excess glucose, insulin instructs your liver to store it as glycogen (the storage-form of glucose, which the liver can release into the blood if your blood sugar levels are low).

The problem arises when your cells stop listening to the signals. This happens when there is too much glucose in your system - for example when you eat a high-sugar diet. The pancreas has to produce more and more insulin to get the glucose out of your blood stream, and over time, cells no longer respond - they become resistant to the insulin's signals.

This creates a two-fold problem. Firstly, insulin resistance means glucose in the bloodstream is not properly absorbed by the cells, creating elevated blood sugar levels: elevated blood sugar causes inflammation. Secondly, high levels of insulin also cause inflammation, which in turn cause hormone imbalances.

This is why many medical professionals believe that insulin resistance can cause PCOS. It therefore makes sense that, since PCOS is triggered by insulin resistance, it can be helped by improving insulin sensitivity.

Insulin resistance also impacts other areas of fertility. Because it disrupts hormone levels, it interferes with how the ovaries release eggs, making it harder for you to conceive. Even if you do conceive, these hormone fluctuations can increase the risk of miscarriage by up to 50%. Insulin resistance is no joke. Suddenly, those sweet treats look a little less appealing. Understanding just how big an impact insulin resistance can have should make any initially difficult food choices a whole lot easier. Giving up some of your favorite foods and working out regularly is a small price to pay for a chance at a healthy, full-term pregnancy.

There are several ways you can test for insulin resistance. The two most common are the fasting blood glucose test and the glucose tolerance test.

A fasting blood glucose test will require you to fast for at least 8 hours prior to the test. A sample of your blood is taken and glucose levels checked. Elevated levels of blood glucose could indicate that the body isn't processing glucose properly, which may indicate insulin resistance. More tests are generally carried out to make sure.

A glucose tolerance test is carried out by taking blood samples before and after drinking a high-glucose solution, to verify how your body is processing glucose. If your blood glucose levels remain high, this is usually a sign of insulin resistance.

Insulin Resistance and Weight Gain

Now we know how insulin resistance works, let's explore its relationship to weight gain.

Weight gain is one of the more noticeable co-conditions with PCOS. Maybe you've had a lifetime of never-ending diets, none of which have worked long term? I know I did. There's a reason for this, and that reason is insulin resistance.

That's not to say no diet will ever work. It's just that most diets do not take insulin resistance into account, and therefore don't hit the mark when it comes to making a significant difference to weight. Don't worry; just because dieting and exercise haven't worked in the past, doesn't mean they won't work now. The trick is to find foods that start helping your body to reverse insulin resistance.

So, why does insulin resistance cause weight gain? As you've learned, insulin signals to your cells to absorb glucose and use it as energy. It also signals to your liver to transform some of that glucose into glycogen; this is a storage form of glucose, which your liver can make use of if your blood sugar levels get too low. But when your glycogen stores are full, your body needs another solution to deal with all that excess glucose. So it signals to your liver again, but this time it asks it to convert the glucose into triglycerides (fats) to be stored in your fat cells.

So you have a situation on your hands: the excess sugar in your diet is not being properly absorbed by your cells, which leads to blood sugar levels becoming elevated and your pancreas releasing a lot of insulin. These high levels of insulin tell your body to store excess glucose as fat, and you gain weight.

This weight gain then exacerbates the problem. Scientists have found that the higher your weight, the more insulin you produce, which makes insulin resistance more likely. It's a vicious circle. There is a debate around whether insulin resistance causes weight gain, or whether weight gain causes insulin resistance. Ultimately, it makes little difference in this context.

The point to remember is that insulin resistance triggers hormone imbalances, increases the risk of miscarriage, and causes weight gain. If you address insulin resistance, you address all these things. And when you address these things, you can begin putting PCOS firmly behind you.

You won't be surprised to know that, since insulin resistance is triggered by an excess of glucose (sugar) in the diet, the changes you need to focus on will center around just that: your diet. What you put on your plate has the power to help you overcome your symptoms and achieve transformational results. That's what this book is all about.

How to Change Your Diet and Exercise Habits

For many women, taking the next proactive step after being diagnosed can be difficult. Symptoms are severe and uncomfortable - missed or irregular periods, excess weight, acne, hirsutism or thinning hair, mood swings - leaving little energy for change. It can feel overwhelming. But it needn't. I'm here to make this new set of healthy habits simple so you can begin your journey to better health.

This section is all about lifestyle changes, especially related to diet and exercise. This is a summary of the information in my first book, which I strongly recommend you check out. It will both serve as an eye-opener and a good foundation for this second installment.

The first thing to remember is that this is NOT YOUR FAULT. So many women feel guilty that they have caused PCOS - but the truth is that we are not taught how to eat well at school, we are not given the right information about diet and exercise. Instead, supermarkets are packed full of high sugar foods (and diet foods are even worse, most of them contain more sugar than the standard versions), and we live lives that are increasingly sedentary. The result: insulin resistance, weight gain, hormone imbalances…. PCOS.

But navigating PCOS lifestyle hacks can be tricky. Should you just focus on losing weight? Is exercise the best way to do this, or diet?

The answer to the weight question is YES. If your BMI (body mass index) is above 25, this indicates you are overweight. Losing weight can significantly improve your symptoms. Not only can it help improve insulin sensitivity, it has also been shown to alleviate depression, another PCOS symptom so many of us struggle with.

But the focal point should not just be losing weight in itself: it should be about gaining health. That means you need to put more emphasis on whole foods, high-protein foods, and healthy fats - we'll explore this in more detail later. While you might be tempted to skip meals in order to lose weight, it is actually important to eat regularly to ensure that your blood sugar levels stay stable. Doing just 30 minutes of exercise a day can prove incredibly beneficial. If you smoke, then it's a good idea to give up - it's no good for your health or your hormones.

Since the main factor that underpins PCOS is insulin resistance, changing what you eat will be the simplest and most effective way to overcome it. The good news is that following a healthier diet (like the one suggested in this book), will improve your health beyond healing PCOS. You'll maintain a stable healthy weight, improve your chances of conceiving, and live longer.

So, if you're ready to show PCOS the door, it's time to dive into the lifestyle strategies that will do just that.

1. Focus on nourishing, not dieting

Following fad diets is the worst thing you can do. Not only is it unsustainable, many diet foods are packed with sugar, which won't help address insulin resistance.

The best way to lose weight and address insulin resistance is to eat a balanced diet that includes plenty of lean protein, healthy fats, complex carbohydrates (more on carbs later), and plenty of antioxidants. By doing this, not only do you maintain healthy blood sugar levels, you also reduce levels of cortisol (a hormone your body produces in response to inflammatory foods and stress).

The easiest way to do this is to fill your shopping basket with plenty of vegetables and leafy greens, fruit, whole grains, beans, nuts and seeds. The recipes in this book will show you how to transform these into tasty meals.

When it comes to protein and fat, the quality is important. Leave vegetable oils and fried foods on the shelf. Healthy sources of fat include avocados, nuts, and seeds. Put that processed meat product down. Healthy sources of protein include beans, legumes, seeds, and organic meat. You'll find antioxidants in all fruits and vegetables, not just the trendy ones like kale. Spices are anti-inflammatory and fantastic sources of antioxidants, so make sure you add them to your day (bonus: they make food taste amazing!).

- Key suggested foods:

Whole foods will be your best friends on this journey: vegetables (kale, zucchini, peppers, radish, broccoli, celery, etc.), fruits (especially berries), whole grains (brown rice, quinoa, buckwheat, millet, couscous, etc.), beans and legumes (lentils, chickpeas, black beans, soy beans, kidney beans, etc.), nuts and seeds (sesame seeds, pumpkin seeds, hemp seeds, chia seeds, flax seeds, almonds, walnuts, cashew nuts, etc.). Start thinking about the types of meals you can make with these foods. Don't worry - you'll find plenty of easy recipes in this book, that will inspire you to get cooking.

2. Cut the crap

The first thing to do to manage your PCOS symptoms is to avoid the foods that cause there to be too much glucose in your blood. What are these foods? Anything made with added sugar or refined carbohydrates (refined carbs include things like white rice, white flour, white pasta - these act like sugar in your body and cause your blood sugar levels to spike). The easiest way to avoid them is to avoid processed foods - cakes, biscuits, dessert pots, ready meals, breakfast cereal, pre-made snacks, all these will have a negative impact on your blood sugar, and cause insulin resistance.

- Key suggested foods:

If you have a sweet tooth, snack of whole fruits instead. While fruit contains sugar (fructose), it also contains fiber and nutrients that slow down the release of glucose in the blood. Make sure you stick with low-sugar fruits such as berries, watermelon, and citrus fruits.

3. Keep your blood sugar balanced

This is where most people get it wrong. You can't just skip breakfast and then grab a sandwich at noon. Not only does this kind of eating pattern make it more likely that you will snack or overeat at mealtimes, it also does nothing to keep your blood sugar level stable.

The better approach is to strike a balance. Instead of fasting for hours and then overeating (hello unstable blood sugar!), aim to schedule and design your meals so they provide energy and nutrients at regular intervals.

- Key suggested foods:

Include healthy sources of both protein and good fats in every meal - this will keep your blood sugar stable while keeping you satisfied and energized until your next meal. A good example of this would be a green smoothie with a vegan protein source (such as kale, apple, soy milk, and hemp seeds).

4. Don't be afraid of fat

Most people think that eating fat will make you fat, but that is inaccurate. It very much depends on the type of fat you eat. While you may be tempted to shy away from fat because you don't want to gain more weight, adding fat to your diet could actually help you shed those extra pounds. In fact, eating healthy fats is an excellent way to keep the body satiated (which means fewer cravings) and, at the same time, help the absorption of vitamins A, D, E, and K (which means lower levels of inflammation and improved hormone levels).

- Key suggested foods:

You will find healthy fats in nuts, seeds, oily fish, olives, avocados and coconuts.

5. Look out for hormone disruptors

Beyond insulin resistance, other aspects of our lifestyle impact hormone levels. Stress, poor quality sleep, and depression all contribute. As do microplastics and pollutants in our air and water.

The solution? To counter stress and depression, give mindfulness and meditation a go. Yoga is a great way to combine mindfulness with a physical practice. Minimize the amount of plastic you come into contact with by using glass bottles and storage jars. Improve your sleep hygiene by setting up a bedtime routine (The PCOS Fix has step by step guidance on how to do this).

- Key suggested foods:

Antioxidant-rich foods will help your body eliminate toxins from pollutants and plastics. These include all fruits and vegetables, but particularly matcha green tea, raw cacao, turmeric, and ginger.

6. Choose your carbs wisely

The type of carbohydrates you consume will either increase insulin resistance, or help reverse it. Don't worry, I'm not about to tell you that carbs are the enemy. However, you must consider the two Q's: quantity and quality. Then, you'll need to think about what you're eating these carbohydrates with.

Let's look at quality first. Forget about refined carbohydrates. These are foods with the protein and fat removed, leaving only the sugars or starch. An example of this is refined flour, which is whole grain flour that has had the bran, germ and endosperm removed. Refined carbohydrates will have the same effect on your body as sugar: quick rise in blood glucose levels. Complex carbohydrates, on the other hand, are your friends. These contain sugars or starches alongside fiber and other nutrients. This fiber slows down the release of glucose, which results in less insulin being needed. Root vegetables, whole grains and beans all contain complex carbohydrates.

Secondly, quantity. No more than a quarter of your plate should be filled with sources of complex carbohydrates. The rest should be made up of mostly low-carb vegetables, alongside a source of protein and some healthy fats.

Thirdly, food pairing. If you pair complex carbs with protein and fat, you slow down the absorption even further. This means you keep your blood glucose stable. Over time, stable blood sugar levels will lead to a normalization of insulin production, which will help you manage and reverse PCOS.

- Key suggested foods:

Some examples of food pairing include: oat crackers (complex carbs) with peanut butter (protein & healthy fats); brown rice (complex carbs), lentils (protein) and toasted almond (healthy fat); wholegrain sourdough bread (complex carbs) with home-made hummus (protein and healthy fats).

7. Eat when your body needs the most energy

When addressing PCOS, it is fundamental that you spread your meals properly throughout the day - this helps you avoid overeating at certain times while undereating at others. It is very common for people to eat lightly in the morning and have a huge dinner at night. That's not ideal! You want to ensure you have your larger meals earlier in the day, and a light meal in the evening so your digestion doesn't stop you from getting a proper night's sleep.

8. Exercise the right way

Dieting is vital, but you cannot overlook the importance of exercise.

Forget intense boot-camp type workout sessions. While they will help you lose weight, they also stress out the body and can do more harm than good. What you need to get rid of PCOS is to build muscle (don't worry, you won't look like a body builder, I promise), because it helps your body to metabolize glucose. You'll also need cardio, because this gets your heart rate up and your body sweating, which is one of the ways your body eliminates toxins (and the more toxins you get rid of, the better for your hormones).

The best type of exercise for PCOS is high intensity interval training (HIIT). During HIIT, you'll alternate working out at high intensity for a short period of time, with working out at lower intensity for a longer time.

Of course, everyone is different, and you will have to adapt your exercise regime to your unique body and needs. Maybe try some different activities and see which one you prefer - after all, exercise also has to be enjoyable, otherwise you will talk yourself out of doing it. Even a brisk walk and some yoga will provide benefits and help your body to deal with PCOS. The trick is to move your body more than you have done in the past.

A Holistic Approach to Managing PCOS

One of the forgotten factors in managing and healing PCOS is stress. If we reduce the stress in our lives, even just a little, we will reap the benefits - not just in terms of feeling calmer, but in terms of better hormone balance.

How? Simple. Take back control. You have full control over your choices. That goes for the food you eat, the amount of exercise you do, but also how you react to the situations that arise in your life.

Interestingly, diet plays a big role in stress. When your blood sugar levels are going up and down like a yoyo, so does your mood. You might also find yourself feeling tired, which will make you feel irritable and frustrated, and attract even more stress into your life. The more stress in your life, the more out of balance your hormones. Stress increases levels of cortisol, which in turn increases inflammation, which in turn exacerbates insulin resistance. This is how even non-diet factors can impact on your body!

So, what can you do? Take a moment to review your life and identify where you feel the most stress, and begin thinking about how you can tackle that situation. Most of the time, it's about learning to say NO to extra commitments while saying YES to more self-care - and by that, I mean saying YES to a whole foods diet, to more time to relax, to doing the things that bring you real joy. It also means taking time to listen to your body - how does it react to the foods you choose?

The more you take control of the parts of your life you have control over, the calmer and more centered you will feel. Don't try to blindly stick to someone else's diet plan - this won't work long term. You have to find the eating pattern that most suits your body. By listening to your body, you can identify what works for you.

My aim is to present you with general, practical guidelines that can help you improve your PCOS symptoms and help you improve your overall health. The following tips will support you to achieve balance in your health and your life.

Make self-care a priority

We are so busy running around for other people that we often forget to make ourselves a priority. And the fact is we need to. It is time to stop putting your needs second. I don't mean that you have to be selfish. In fact, self-care is ultimately an unselfish act. After all, the healthier and happier you are, the more positive an impact you can have.

Often, stress comes from feeling that we don't have any spare time. Carve out that time. The way I did this in my own life was to create a morning routine that gave me that essential "me time." This created a calm mental space from which it was so much easier to stick to healthy habits. How can you give yourself that time to just be, every day? Look at your diary and find moments when you can do that. Whether it's an afternoon reading a book, a relaxing evening bath, or simply a 5-minute meditation, schedule this self-care and stick to it.

These moments will give you a chance to recharge your batteries and fully relax. When you do, your body can spend time repairing and rebalancing.

A simple daily practice: Deep breathing

The simplest yet most ignored tool for managing insulin resistance is stress reduction. Okay, it isn't easy to banish stress from our lives. It is everywhere. Our phones are beeping every minute, we have bills to pay, we have to queue for everything, there are all of these things competing for our attention. How can you center yourself in the middle of all this?

As basic as it might sound, we need to return to the breath. If you have ever been to a yoga class, you probably noticed how often your instructor stressed the importance of breathing. The simple practice of deep breathing engages your parasympathetic nervous system - your body's "rest and digest" mode. Here, things slow down and you are able to remain calm in response to any stress. As opposed to our "fight or flight" mode, which happens when we react to stress. When we're in fight or flight mode, our cortisol levels shoot up, and our hormones suffer. What's more, cortisol disrupts our appetite signals, which makes it harder to eat sensibly.

Next time you feel stressed, take a moment to consciously take a long, slow, deep breath. Feel the air expand your stomach, and send your belly button towards your spine as you exhale. This will clear your mind and relax you as you plan your next move. The more you can pause for a few seconds instead of instantly reacting to external stressors, the easier it will become. As you spend more time in a calm space, your body can spend time rebalancing and healing itself.

Planning ahead

I've asked you to schedule in some self-care. Planning is also essential when you transition to a healthier diet. Plan your menu for the week, and then write up your shopping list, schedule when you can do some meal preparation, and so forth. Once you've done that, plan when you will exercise. It can either be a regular routine, for example 20 minutes of high intensity interval training every morning, or you can change it up, for example a brisk walk on Monday afternoon, a yoga class on Tuesday, swimming on Wednesday and so on - what matters if you are moving your body and engaging your muscles.

Don't aim for perfection

Aiming for perfection only leads to one place: stress. The best way to approach these changes is with an 80/20 approach. Nutrition does not have to be restrictive. Indeed, when it is, it only creates cravings (if you're told you can't have chocolate, you will only think of chocolate) and potential imbalances (for example, a strict raw food diet can lack essential nutrients). What's more, we all respond differently to foods.

The thing to remember is balance. This is about what works for you, while following the basic principles of a PCOS-friendly diet (one that balances blood sugar and therefore redresses insulin resistance). The 80/20 approach means you stick with your healthy habits 80% of the time, allowing for the occasional deviation. For example, sharing a slice of cake when you meet up with a friend, or having a glass of wine on Friday night. This is about reducing stress levels, not creating a life where you can't enjoy yourself.

Part of the 80/20 approach is also not beating yourself up for where you are right now. Keep your focus on where you're heading with these changes. Maybe your goal is a healthy pregnancy. Or perhaps you just yearn to have a normal cycle, to clear up your skin, to feel healthy again. Whatever it is, that journey begins with accepting how you are in this moment, and pledging to love yourself enough to make changes.

Nobody is perfect and I do not expect you to have a perfect diet since it doesn't exist. What matters is that you listen to your body and give it what it needs: a whole foods diet, some daily movement, and a little love in the form of self-care. How that looks is up to you, and how you find out what works is by trying different things, like the ones I've outlined in this book. As you do, you will come to discover what makes you feel good, and you'll be able to strike that right balance.

CHAPTER TWO:

INTRODUCING THE INSULIN RESISTANT DIET FOR PCOS

Ever since I was diagnosed with PCOS, I have been determined to write a cookbook to support other women in their healing journey. More important than bringing new foods into our diet or eliminating old ones, it is more about creating new, healthy habits that you can stick with in the long term.

I believe there is no point in creating another generic cookbook, when we both know that you don't have space in your kitchen for another cooking gadget and you don't have time to spend four hours every night cooking a meal. That is why I created this guide. It is aimed at the busy professional, the creative artist, and the woman who simply hates cooking - you're all welcome here! This isn't about being an expert chef, it's about cooking healthy, simple foods that make a real difference to your health.

Some foods are well worth incorporating in your diet, particularly for their impact on PCOS symptoms. On the flip side, there are several "no-go" foods that we need to eliminate, because they can aggravate symptoms. Before we get into some tasty recipes for every time of day - breakfast, lunch, dinner, and healthy snacks - let's discuss the must-haves and the must-not-haves in more detail.

Superfoods

How amazing would it be to have a list of foods that help your PCOS symptoms? Well, there is: my PCOS superfoods list! Make sure you have at least one item off the list every day.

Berries

Berries are a great substitute for all that processed sugar. They taste delicious and have plenty of natural fruity sweetness. Unlike sugar, berries actually support your health because they are packed with antioxidants. What's more, the fiber in berries slows down the absorption of sugar, making them a strong ally in the crusade against insulin resistance and a life-saver in curbing those sugar cravings.

Avocados

Whether it is avocado on toast or a super healthy guacamole dip for game night, avocados are renowned for being brain-food. They're a great source of omega-3 and vitamin E, both of which give skin a healthy glow. The unsaturated fats in avocado help regulate hormone imbalances and irregular periods, as well as balance blood sugar and reduce inflammation - exactly the areas that you want to focus on when healing PCOS. There are many ways you can include avocados in your diet: chop them into salads, mash them into guacamole, blend them into creamy sauces or even turn them into chocolate mousse!

Nuts and Seeds

Nuts and seeds excellent for keeping you full and regulating sugar levels, so you might find it helpful to always have some nuts and seeds on hand for when you fancy a snack, especially during the first week of your transition. A handful of trail mix (not the shop-bought kind with dried fruit or added sugar) might prove very useful when you feel your energy crashing at the office. Nuts can help reduce levels of male hormones, while seeds (such as flax seeds or chia seeds) help your body detoxify thanks to their high fiber content.

Cinnamon

Cinnamon helps regulate blood sugar and it is a tasty addition to meals, particularly breakfasts and snacks. The data around cinnamon's ability to regulate blood sugar is extraordinary: it can actually lower blood sugar levels by up to 29%. This is just one of the benefits. It also has anti-inflammatory properties and may lower the risk of heart disease. Cinnamon contains powerful antioxidants, which help lower inflammation and strengthen the immune system. Comforting and slightly sweet, it's well worth adding a sprinkle of cinnamon to your meals.

What to Eat to Improve Your PCOS Symptoms

We know PCOS goes hand in hand with hormone imbalances and metabolism problems. But it's also related to numerous health complications, such as diabetes, cardiovascular disorders, and an increased chance of endometrial cancer. Research shows that a healthy diet can help alleviate all of these health risks.

The Relationship Between Diet And PCOS

There are many ways in which diet affects PCOS and I have touched on this in The PCOS Fix, which I strongly recommend that you read if you haven't already. When we look at how diet affects PCOS, we keep coming back to the importance of managing body weight and insulin resistance.

We've seen that insulin resistance is a significant factor in PCOS and its many symptoms. When insulin is brought in balance with the right PCOS diet, symptoms are improved, making the condition less severe. This is important, because insulin resistance can lead to the development of type 2 diabetes and obesity. However, if you follow a diet that provides the body with all essential nutrients, while keeping blood sugar balanced and insulin production under control, you can reduce your symptoms and feel better.

Foods That Improve PCOS

What you decide to include on your plate has a significant effect on your PCOS symptoms. But, as I have stressed in other parts of this book, there is no one-size-fits-all diet for this condition. There are, however, three recognized diets that help improve symptoms.

The Low Glycemic Index (GI) Diet

Foods with a lower GI are generally digested more slowly thanks to their fiber, protein and healthy fat content, so they do not cause a spike in insulin levels, unlike foods with a high GI (such as refined carbohydrates). A low GI diet includes plenty of vegetables and leafy vegetables, like kale, as well as beans and legumes, whole grains, nuts and seeds. The thing to remember is low-carb and minimally processed foods.

An Anti-Inflammatory Diet

This type of diet focuses on limiting the amount of inflammatory foods on your plate, while filling up on foods that actively fight inflammation, such as berries, fresh and leafy vegetables, turmeric, and omega-3.

Since inflammation can exacerbate PCOS symptoms and even lead to hormone imbalances, the anti-inflammatory diet is a good option to try. Bonus: it will help reduce other inflammation-related symptoms such as weight-gain, extreme fatigue, cravings, and irritability.

The DASH Diet

DASH stands for dietary approaches to stop hypertension, and is recommended for people at risk of heart disease or stroke.

But it has also proven beneficial in the management of PCOS symptoms. The DASH diet reduces the amount of saturated fats and added sugars on your plate. It centers around vegetables, fruit, fish, poultry, whole grains, and low-fat dairy products. Following a well-planned DASH diet is a sure way to reduce insulin resistance and belly fat.

The interesting thing to note about these three diets, and indeed most healthy diets, is that they center around common principles: the avoidance of processed foods and the focus on whole, unprocessed, natural foods.

A diet designed to reduce PCOS symptoms should include the following:

- Whole, natural, plant-based foods (minimally processed, without added sugars)
- Vegetables (kale, spinach, zucchini, peppers, etc.)
- Fruit (especially berries)
- Legumes and beans (chickpeas, lentils, kidney beans, black beans, soy beans, etc.)
- Healthy fats (avocado, olive oil, and coconut oil)
- Natural spices and herbs (like turmeric and cinnamon, parsley and cilantro)
- Nuts and seeds (almonds, walnuts, pumpkin seeds, flax seeds, etc.)
- Fatty fish (tune, sardines, salmon)

Regardless of which diet you choose to follow, losing weight can significantly improve your PCOS symptoms. Focusing on plant sources of fats, minimizing your reliance on animal products, and piling your plate high with fiber-rich vegetables and fruits, will help you lose weight. Reducing your intake of carbohydrates and favoring sources of complex carbohydrates will also help improve your metabolism, lower cholesterol levels, and reduce the risk of chronic diseases like heart disease and diabetes. On a closer-to-home level, these types of diet will help regularize your periods, clear up your skin, stabilize your mood, and improve your overall quality of life.

Foods to Avoid with PCOS

Now that we have covered some of the best foods to manage PCOS symptoms, it is time to turn to the foods you must say goodbye to.

When you first get started on your PCOS journey, it is enough to make small changes. But I have to be really honest. Eating kale is great, but if you're still indulging in high-sugar foods and drinks, it just won't make a difference. To heal PCOS you need to both add (foods that redress the imbalances) and remove (foods that cause the imbalances).

Don't worry - for every food we are removing, we are adding something else. I'll share my favorite healthy alternatives so you don't need to feel like you're missing out.

Sugar

We are eating way too much sugar. We're addicted to the stuff. And it is killing us. Not only does it cause weight gain, it increases inflammation, disrupts your hormones, and increases the risk of depression. Not so sweet after all!

The main problem with sugar is how it affects our insulin levels. Sugary foods cause a huge increase in blood glucose (blood sugar high), which the body then has to deal with through insulin (blood sugar low). These blood sugar highs and lows don't just cause your emotions to be all over the place, they also lead to overeating, which leads to you putting more weight on. It's a negative cycle.

There are two main types of sugar in our diet: glucose and fructose. Glucose, in adequate amounts, is not harmful. In fact, your body converts carbohydrates into glucose because this is your cells preferred form of fuel. Fructose is another story. The fructose that is naturally present in fruit is fine - it is accompanied by fiber and vitamins, which means the body can process it. However, fructose in a processed form, for example high fructose corn syrup, is hard for the body to deal with. Fructose is not your cells' preferred source of fuel and is therefore processed differently: it is metabolized (broken down) by the liver. Over time, this can stress the liver out. Since the liver produces many hormones, this is bad news for PCOS sufferers. Fructose also disrupts hunger and satiety signals, which can lead to over-eating.

The other problem with sugar is that it is literally everywhere. In almost all processed foods - even the savory ones. To stop eating sugar, you must leave those foods on the shelf. It sounds challenging, but once you start, you'll wonder what took you so long.

When you cut sugar out of your diet, you will see significant weight loss. And while you may experience some unwanted emotional symptoms during the first few days, if you stick with it, you'll transform your relationship with food. Think about it: if you eat foods that cause you to overeat, you lose touch with your natural appetite. By choosing natural, whole foods, you reconnect with this part of yourself. It's empowering.

As you begin to cut sugar out of your life, keep a journal of how you feel emotionally and physically. Writing things down will help you cope with the cravings, and you'll be able to see, black on white, how much better you feel without added sugar in your life. Trust me, you are sweet enough.

Healthier alternatives to sweet treats:

- An apple and a handful of toasted almonds
- A bowl of berries with toasted coconut flakes and full-fat organic yogurt

- Home-made trail mix
- Dark chocolate

Carbohydrates

Don't worry. Like I said before, you don't have to give up all carbs forever. But you do need to significantly reduce the quantity, and shift the type of carbohydrates you're eating.

Sure, these changes won't be a walk in the park - but anything worth having requires a little work. Isn't your health worth it? All I ask is that you try it just for 30 days - if you don't feel significant improvements, I will be the first one to admit defeat and pass you a bag of chips!

When I started looking at how to reduce my carbohydrate intake, the first thing that shocked me was just how much of my diet was made up of carbohydrates! I was aware that sugary snacks and soda weren't good for my health, and I knew they had to go. It was harder, however, to consider removing carbs. And it was difficult at the time to know what I would replace them with.

Thankfully, there are plenty of delicious alternatives. Once I started on my journey of no gluten and minimal carbs, I felt like I was eating real food for the very first time. I was so used to feeling over-full after every meal but being hungry a relatively short time later. Food-derived energy was a transient commodity for me and if I didn't capture that 30 minutes after a meal when I was able to concentrate, I would be chasing it for the rest of the day with sugary drinks and chocolate bars. Maybe this is a pattern you recognize? Switching to healthier complex carbohydrates was a total game changer.

When I think of my past diet, I am shocked at how it overtook my daily life. I thought cooking and preparing healthy food in advance would take up so much time, but what I quickly found was that it didn't take up as much time as I was already spending being distracted by how hungry I was, popping to the store to stock up on afternoon sugar, or sitting at my desk trying not to fall asleep as the dreaded 'afternoon slump' hit me. It turns out that taking a few hours out of every week to prepare healthy meals is nothing compared to the hours I was wasting every day trying to keep up with the chronic game of catch up that my body was playing with my sugar levels.

So, remove refined carbohydrates from your life: no more white bread, white pasta, white rice, sugar, fizzy drinks, pre-made treats and desserts.

Instead, fill up on healthy sources of complex carbohydrates; replace your usual carb with something more nutrient dense and transform your meal into a PCOS-busting alternative. For example, use brown rice instead of couscous, or sweet potato wedges instead of French fries.

Other sources of complex carbohydrates include:

- Root vegetables (carrots, sweet potatoes, celeriac, parsnip, beetroot…)
- Whole grains (brown rice, millet, quinoa, buckwheat…)
- Beans and legumes (lentils, chickpeas, black beans, pinto beans, kidney beans, adzuki beans, mung beans…)
- Nuts and seeds (almonds, walnuts, brazil nuts, pumpkin seeds, sunflower seeds, chia seeds, flax seeds…)

Processed Foods

There are several problems with processed foods, beyond their sugar content. For one, they can contain trans-saturated fats. Trans-fats cause weight gain and increase inflammation - two factors in PCOS. They're so unhealthy that the FDA has banned the addition of trans-fats in food from 2018 - however, food manufacturers are still able to sell food containing trans-fats until 2020, so make sure you check the label and avoid anything containing hydrogenated or partially hydrogenated oils.

The other issue with processed foods is that they contain other artificial additives - whether that's preservatives, flavor enhancers or colors - that do not belong in the body.

Just think about the process of processed food for a moment. It is put together in factories, using artificial ingredients so the food lasts longer on the shelf. It's then stored in plastic containers until you buy it and place it in a microwave to be radiated at extreme temperatures (which leaches some of the plastic from the container into the food itself). How nutritious is this food? Also, how tasty is it really? Judging by the amount of extra salt in most ready-meals, I'd say not really. Home cooked food is so much better. Ready meals may feel convenient, but in the long term they rob you of your health. I don't know about you, but I'd rather spend a little time in the kitchen, and protect my health.

In the next few chapters, I will show you how to incorporate fresh food and healthy eating into your day. Regardless of your schedule, there are always alternatives to eating ready meals and sugary snacks. This will not just reduce your PCOS symptoms, but also help cultivate good gut health and ward off other more serious health problems. The more we focus on natural foods, the better our bodies feel!

Gluten and Dairy

I'm going to cover both gluten and dairy together because, although they are different types of food, and appear in vastly different forms in your diet, the reason why you should cut them out is the same: both these foods cause inflammation, and both these foods impact on your gut health... and both these things worsen PCOS symptoms like acne.

First thing to note is just how prevalent both these foods are in our diets. You've probably eaten them every day, for years. We add dairy to breakfast cereal and pour it in coffee, there is gluten in every slice of bread or cake, every pastry. But that's not all - because both gluten and diary are cheap fillers, they are added to many processed foods, even those you wouldn't think of - another reason to cut processed foods out of your diet. For example, many supermarket breads contain dehydrated milk powder.

Putting aside the social and environmental impact of dairy, which I'm not going to go into in this book, let's focus on the health concerns. Most people do not have enough lactase (a digestive enzyme responsible for breaking down lactose - the sugar in milk) to properly digest dairy after childhood. Indeed, we are the only species of animal to consume milk beyond infancy (and indeed, to consume milk from another species). What's more, studies have found that drinking milk causes a huge spike in insulin - the very thing we want to avoid! As if that wasn't enough, conventionally produced milk contains antibiotic residues, and these disrupt your gut bacteria, leading to, you guessed it, inflammation. Other issues surrounding dairy is that it is mucus-forming; you might have noticed that you have a stuffy or runny nose when you eat it - or maybe this is such an everyday occurrence that you no longer notice. Regardless, you'll definitely notice an improvement when you give dairy a miss for a couple of weeks!

When it comes to gluten, again we're eating way too much. But there are other issues too - for example, the fact that the most commonly used varieties of wheat contain more gluten protein than they used to. Gluten is an anti-nutrient, and the immune system tends to react to it as it would to an intruder: by attacking it. How? Through inflammation. So, every time you eat gluten, your immune system reacts. Naturally, this stresses the body. How can it focus on balancing hormones and keeping you healthy if it is constantly having to fight with the foods you choose?

Many women with PCOS are sensitive to gluten and dairy without realizing it, and notice significant weight loss and health improvements after cutting them out. Doesn't that motivate you to give these two foods a miss?

When I first learned that I had PCOS, I had already been thinking about trying a vegan lifestyle. My diagnosis was the push I needed to go for it. The potential health benefits and reduction of my PCOS symptoms far outweighed the convenience of carrying on with my eating habits. I'm so glad I made the choice to move to a plant-based diet, free from both dairy and gluten.

You can do it too, and you will feel fantastic when you do. If you're feeling overwhelmed, then don't try to remove everything at once. Take it one step at a time. Cut out gluten from your diet for 30 days and see how you feel, and then cut out dairy for 30 days. Track your progress in your journal - this will help keep you motivated.

The other thing to remember is that you have options. Milk may be off the menu, but you'll be happy to know there are plant-based alternatives that taste much better than dairy. And when it comes to gluten-free grains, you are spoilt for choice these days - you can find pasta made from beans and breads made from seeds in most health food shops (just make sure you check the label and choose those made with only whole, natural ingredients).

In the next few chapters, you'll find my favorite gluten-free, dairy-free, plant-based meals, and the

30-Day PCOS Boot Camp so you can start putting your new diet into practice.

Processed Meat

This is a totally taboo topic, but I'll address it now, before we get into recipes. As I've said, I am completely vegan. I decided to switch because meat causes inflammation, and inflammation doesn't do your PCOS any good.

But I understand that not everyone is ready to make that change. If you're not, consider at least the quality and quantity of the meat you consume.

Let's address quality first. Conventionally produced meat comes from cows that have been fed poor quality feed (including genetically modified grains, the remains of other cattle, and plastic pellets), as well as antibiotics (both because these make the animals fatter, but also because of the unsanitary conditions in feedlots and slaughterhouses). The result is a food that can potentially cause gut inflammation, while putting the immune system under strain. The World Health Organization has classified red meat as "probably carcinogenic to humans" (Group 2A carcinogen), while processed meat (things like sandwich meats, sausages, ham, corned beef, etc.) as "carcinogenic to humans" (Group 1 carcinogen - tobacco is in this group).

What about quantity? Never before have we eaten so much meat. It used to be a bit of a treat, something one would have once a week, maybe even less. Now, we're encouraged to eat meat several times a day, sometimes even two or three different types of meat in one dish. Not only is this not sustainable for our planet, which is already struggling to cope with our modern way of life, it is not sustainable for health. We are not designed to consume this much animal protein - our health suffers as a consequence.

Begin transitioning to a more plant-based diet by deciding that at least one of your meals will be vegan, every day. Then, go further, make it two meals. Before you know it, you'll wonder how you ate so much meat in the first place. We are conditioned into thinking that we need meat for protein, but the truth is there is as much protein in plant foods, for example quinoa, buckwheat, hemp seeds and soy - all of which are as protein-dense as meat, with the added benefit that they contain gut-friendly fiber!

While you transition, start reviewing the kind of meat you buy. Go to your local butcher, ask how the animal was treated, what it was fed, and choose organic, sustainably produced, humanely raised meat, poultry, and eggs. When it comes to fish, avoid farmed fish (which also contain antibiotic residues), and go for wild caught instead.

Caffeine and Alcohol

I've included these two together to minimize discomfort…. you might want to brace yourself for this one! Yes, you will have to remove most of the caffeine and alcohol from your life. Why? Because both of them stress out your body and can exacerbate PCOS symptoms.

Your liver processes alcohol like a toxin, which means it has less energy to produce sex hormones (one of the problems with PCOS). Caffeine can stress your adrenal glands, increasing your levels of cortisol - and excess cortisol can increase inflammation.

Believe me when I say: I know how difficult this is. If you come from a small town like me, you will know just how important a few drinks are to lubricate social occasions, and there is nothing like a hot cup of coffee to get the day started. And, full disclosure, I have both caffeine and alcohol, in moderation. I still enjoy a morning coffee while writing my journal, but I stop at one. And I do have the occasional glass of wine, but, again, I do stop at one…well, maybe two. But when I first started, I knew I had to completely overhaul my life so I cut both out completely for around two years. And I can honestly say that I have never felt better. Again here, don't panic. Think 80/20 and think quality. If you have one organic coffee a day, and one or two glasses of organic red wine a week, as part of a healthy whole-foods diet, that is just fine.

It is the same as when you stop eating sugar and find that your energy levels regulate themselves. When I stopped drinking alcohol and caffeine, I found that my sleep cycle normalized, I was better able to concentrate, and I could manage my mood and my emotions much better. And it wasn't until I went back through my journal entries that I realized just how significant this shift was. I even started my days earlier, as the quality of my sleep had improved to the stage where I did not need to sleep as long, and I was waking up without an alarm, ready to take on the day.

This might not seem possible to you and, depending on your lifestyle, you might not even want to consider giving up these little pleasures. I completely understand. But remember what you're trying to achieve: radical health transformation, improved fertility, and no more PCOS symptoms. That involves change. If you're sick of PCOS affecting your ability to live your life on your terms, then you will find the strength to make changes in your life. I believe in you. You must also believe in yourself.

CHAPTER THREE:

MY FAVORITE BREAKFAST RECIPES

Breakfast can be a key time to nourish yourself, and be ready to face the day. If you have been following along with The PCOS Fix, you may have adopted a new morning routine, which means by the time you come to try these recipes, you will have already been out for a walk, meditated, journaled, and not looked at your smartphone once...right?

But even if you're not having superhero mornings just yet, you can still set up your day for success. When you are planning to cook breakfast in the morning, it is a good idea to start preparing the night before - for example by pre-chopping some vegetables, or even making some of the elements in advance. If you plan your weekly meals on a Sunday, you can do your grocery shopping once a week and then schedule time to prepare meals. Placing this schedule on your fridge is a good way of keeping it fresh in your mind.

So, by the time it comes to the morning, I am assuming that you know what you are cooking, you have the ingredients ready, and that you have set aside enough time to be able to complete the recipe without getting stressed out. Try these recipes on the weekend first; after you've done them once or twice, they will be even quicker to make!

We'll start with a good old-fashioned smoothie recipe, but with a bit of a twist - vegetable smoothies are a much healthier way to start your day, and will deliver all those leafy greens that you need to fight inflammation. There is minimal prep, zero waste, and absolutely no excuse not to prepare this fresh - you can even drink it on your way to work. If your mornings really are too intense, you can prepare your smoothie the night before, keep it chilled in the fridge, and drink it the next day.

Remember the advice on plastics from my first book, and make sure that you store your smoothie in either a glass or metal container, or at the very least one that's BPA-free.

KALE AND SPINACH KICKSTARTER

There is literally no better way to kickstart your day than with a large smoothie, packed full of healing veggies and bursting with vitamins and minerals. One of my personal favorites is this kale and spinach smoothie, and it is so simple to make.

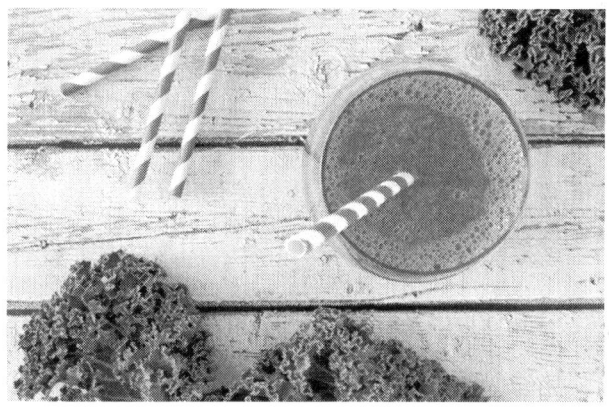

Ingredients (serves 1):

- 1 apple (cored and sliced)
- 1 banana (peeled)
- 1 handful of kale (freshly washed)
- 1 handful of spinach (freshly washed)
- ½ cup of cold water or ice chips
- ¼-inch piece ginger root (peeled)
- 1 tbsp chia seeds

Method:

1. The main thing to remember when making smoothies is that you need a healthy base, but at the same time it needs to taste good. Adding an apple and banana will give it a sweetness which balances out the bitterness of the kale and the ginger.
2. Place all the ingredients in your blender, adding the greens last.
3. Blend until smooth - you may need to push down the greens using your blender's tamper stick.
4. Pour into a glass and enjoy immediately.

Handy Tips

Ginger is a superfood. Not only is it anti-inflammatory, but it helps you stave off hunger throughout the day.

As you get more comfortable with making smoothies, you'll soon be freestyling your own. For example:

- Add a couple of tablespoons of vegan protein powder
- Add a tablespoon of hemp seeds or chia seeds (extra protein and healthy fats)
- Swap the spinach or kale for cucumber or zucchini

- Add a squeeze of lime
- Add a pear instead of an apple

Having a green smoothie in the morning with some shaved ginger will help you get used to eating later in the day. You'll have more energy - maybe even enough energy for a morning workout! This will help you as you go through the 30-Day Boot Camp because you will slowly put back the time at which you begin eating - by reducing your eating window, you give your body time in the fasted state, helping get your cravings under control. It also helps with self-healing and allows the body time to regenerate and balance hormones.

Of course, there will be days when you want a hearty breakfast, so check out the next few recipes for filling breakfasts that will keep you energized till lunchtime.

SHAKSHUKA

Shakshuka offers a nice twist to how you might usually eat eggs in the morning. This North African dish is packed with healthy fats, protein, and antioxidants. It's pretty quick and simple to make too, and is baked in the oven (giving you time to get dressed or write in your journal as the eggs cook).

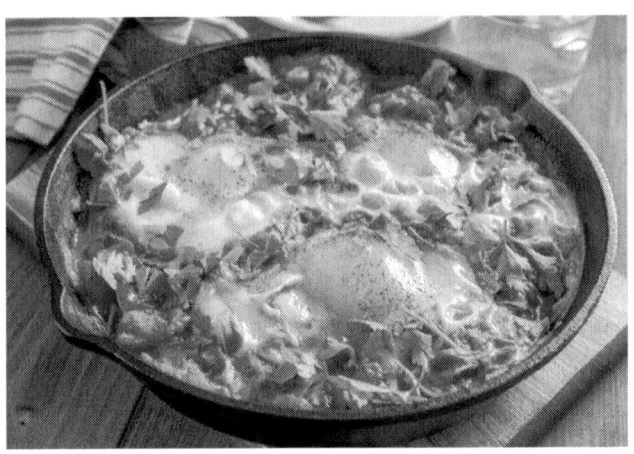

Ingredients (serves 2):
- 4 large organic free-range eggs
- 1 can of chopped tomatoes or 4 fresh medium-sized tomatoes (chopped)
- 1 large onion (chopped)
- 2 bell peppers (sliced finely)
- 1 tbsp tomato paste

- 2 tbsp cold water
- 1 pinch cayenne pepper
- 1 clove garlic (minced or crushed)
- 3 tbsp olive oil
- Salt and pepper to taste

Method:

1. You will need a skillet or a frying pan that can be used for both frying and oven baking.
2. Preheat your oven to 350F.
3. Finely dice the onion and garlic.
4. Heat the olive oil in the pan, and add the onion and garlic. Lightly sauté until the onions are translucent.
5. Add the tomatoes, cayenne pepper, bell peppers, and water, and cook until the mixture begins to bubble.
6. With a wooden spoon, create four small holes in the mixture. Crack an egg into each hole.
7. Place the pan in the pre-heated oven and bake for 10 to 15 minutes, depending how runny or hard you like your yolks.
8. Remove from the oven, season with salt and pepper, and enjoy. It can also be served for brunch or lunch.

Handy Tips

You can have fun with this recipe by adding different flavors and vegetables.

- Add a tbsp of ras el hanout spice for a more pronounced depth of flavor.
- Add mushrooms instead of peppers.
- Add a cup of chopped cooked sweet potatoes for an even heartier dish.

PROTEIN BOX

When it comes to sticking to a healthy regime, you don't want to be running out of the door without having had a proper breakfast and then have to pick something up on the way to work. The protein box will be your best friend here - both for breakfast on the go, or as a protein-packed lunch. Here's one of my favorite combinations!

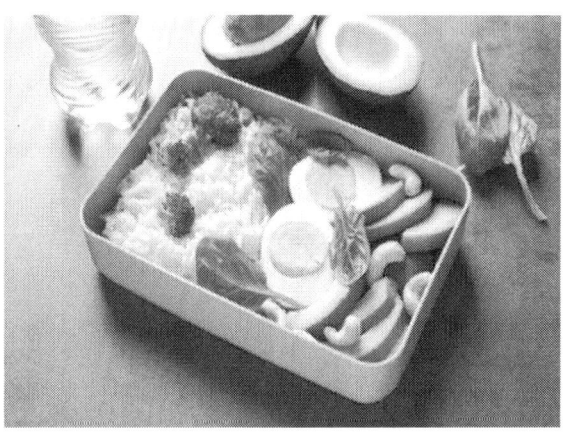

Ingredients (serves 1):

- 2 hard-boiled eggs
- 1 handful freshly washed spinach
- 1 avocado (sliced)
- 1/2 cup cooked brown rice
- 2 tbsp pine nuts
- 1-2 tbsp tamari soy sauce

Method:

1. Place all the ingredients in your lunch container. Keep in the fridge until you're ready to eat.
2. Perfect option to make the day before, if you know you have a busy morning ahead.

Handy Tips

This protein box is perfect for lunch or for breakfast - it is the adult equivalent of packing a sandwich in your lunchbox the night before school. Except that, unlike a sandwich, the nutrients in this protein box will keep you satisfied till your next meal. Protein is both filling and energizing, so you might find you have much more energy than you used to! You can easily prepare the ingredients for protein boxes and assemble two or three in advance.

Why not make up your own protein box with different ingredients?

- You can replace the eggs with 1/2 cup of tofu, tempeh, or beans.
- Try kale instead of spinach.
- Have quinoa, buckwheat, or millet instead of rice.
- Replace the pine nuts for pumpkin seeds or sunflower seeds.
- Swap the soy sauce for coconut aminos, or a mix of sesame oil and lemon juice.

HOME-MADE
PROTEIN-PACKED GRANOLA

You know those mornings when all you fancy is a bowl of cereal? Most supermarket versions contain crazy amounts of sugar and therefore aren't a good option. What if you could make your very own granola, packed with protein and complex carbohydrates? Both xylitol and chicory root syrup are low-carb sweeteners that deliver sweetness without spiking your insulin levels. Serve this granola with organic yogurt, coconut yogurt, or even on top of a smoothie.

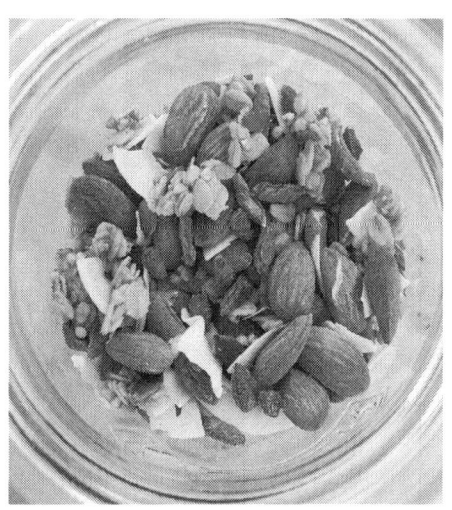

Ingredients:

- 1 cup gluten-free oats
- 1 cup buckwheat grots (unroasted)
- 1/2 cup pumpkin seeds
- 1/2 cup sunflower seeds
- 1/2 cup cashew nuts (roughly chopped)
- 1 tbsp coconut flour
- 3 tbsp coconut oil
- 1/4 cup xylitol (or you can use chicory root syrup)
- 1/2 tsp cinnamon
- 1/4 tsp vanilla extract (optional)
- 1 handful of goji berries and coconut flakes (optional)

Method:

1. Preheat your oven to 350F.
2. Melt the coconut oil, set aside.
3. In large bowl, place the oats, buckwheat, nuts, seeds, coconut flour, xylitol, cinnamon and vanilla extract, and mix to combine.
4. Add the coconut oil and mix well.
5. Pour onto an oven tray lined with baking paper, and bake for 10-14 minutes, or until golden.
6. Allow to cool completely, add a handful of goji berries and coconut flakes (optional - this makes a great trail mix) then store in an airtight container - it will keep for 2-3 weeks.

Handy Tips

If you always have healthy snacks on hand, you can easily stick to new habits. A handful of this granola with a piece of fruit makes for a satisfying snack. And you can mix it up to create different flavors.

- Use almonds instead of cashew nuts.
- Add a teaspoon of turmeric powder, or
- Add a tablespoon or two of cacao powder.

MEXICAN BLACK BEAN CHILI

This black bean chili is a delicious breakfast. It tastes great when cooked fresh, but also makes a tasty leftover - perfect for those days when you just can't be bothered to cook. Add a vegan sausage and you've got yourself a nutritious, filling and warming meal.

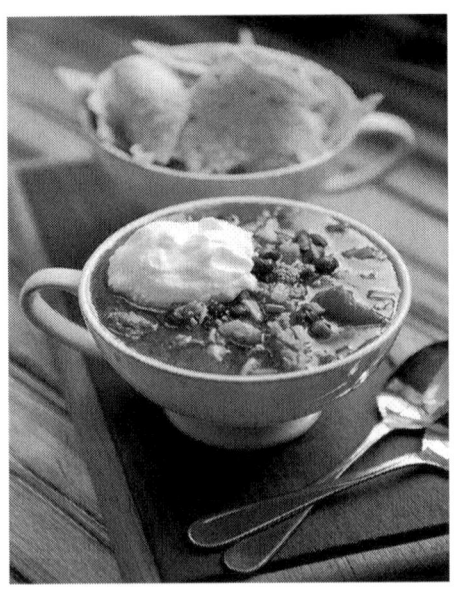

Ingredients (serves 4):

- 2 tbsp olive oil
- 2 tsp paprika
- 1 tsp ground cumin

- 1/2 tsp dried oregano
- 2 onions (finely chopped)
- 1 tbsp minced garlic
- 1 chipotle chili (optional - omit if you don't like too much heat)
- 2 cans of cooked black beans (rinsed and drained)
- 1 cup vegetable stock
- 2 cans chopped tomatoes
- 1/4 cup lime juice
- A handful of chopped cilantro
- A spoonful of coconut yogurt, to serve

Method:

1. In a large pan, heat the olive oil, and cook the onions and garlic until the onion is almost translucent. Add the paprika, cumin and oregano, and cook for a few minutes, taking care not to burn the spices.
2. Add the beans, vegetable stock, and chopped tomatoes to the pan. Heat until the mixture begins to bubble.
3. Reduce heat to simmer, and cook until it begins to thicken - around 15-25 minutes.
4. While that is cooking, cook the vegan sausages as per packet instructions.
5. To serve, spoon the chili into a bowl, stir in some lime juice and chopped cilantro, and top with a

bit of yogurt and a couple of vegan sausages. Breakfast has never been so epic - and it works as a tasty dinner as well!

Handy Tips

Chili is a great option if you're looking for something spicy. But, if you don't like spicy food, you can leave out the chipotle chili. You can bulk up the dish by adding other vegetables.

- Use kidney beans or turtle beans instead of black beans.
- Try replacing the paprika, cumin and oregano with a mild curry spice mix.
- Use coconut oil instead of olive oil.
- Add mushrooms, diced sweet potatoes, or diced eggplant for a more complete meal.

SCRAMBLED TOFU

Who says you can't have eggs when you go vegan? Ok, you can't have eggs, but you can have scrambled tofu instead. Fluffy, satisfying and flavorsome, this makes the perfect breakfast. Tofu is packed with protein and healthy fiber to keep you full up till lunch.

Ingredients (serves 2):

- 8oz firm tofu
- 1 tbsp olive oil
- 2 tbsp nutritional yeast
- 1/2 tsp turmeric powder
- 1/2 tsp paprika powder
- 1/2 tsp garlic powder
- 1/4 tsp onion powder
- 1/3 cup oat cream or soy milk
- 1/4 tsp black salt (gives the tofu an eggy flavor - optional)

Method:

1. In a bowl, mash the tofu with a fork until it is roughly broken up.
2. In a small bowl, whisk together the oat cream, nutritional yeast, turmeric, paprika, garlic powder, onion powder until well combined.

3. In a frying pan, heat the olive oil, add the tofu and fry on medium heat for 2-3 minutes.
4. Add the sauce and stir to distribute evenly. Keep cooking for a few minutes, until the tofu has absorbed some of the sauce. Stir in the black salt, if using, and serve.

Handy Tips:

- Don't have onion or garlic powder? No problem - swap for mild curry powder instead.
- Add spring onions, mushrooms, and finely diced peppers to the tofu for added fiber and nutrients.
- Serve your scrambled tofu with avocado and roasted tomatoes for an epic brunch plate.
- Add scrambled tofu to your lunchtime power bowls (more on these in the next chapter!).

CHAPTER FOUR:

MY FAVORITE LUNCH RECIPES

Sure, it would be easy for me to create gourmet lunch recipes and fill a whole book with mouth-watering creations that take hours to prepare. But, realistically, if your lunchtime is anything like mine, you are looking for recipes that are simple, quick to make, and can be eaten cold.

Leftovers may not be glamorous, but they are very tasty and a good solution for those of us who are pressed for time. What's more, this saves you money since you minimize any food waste, and don't need to buy lunch outside. For example, say you make roasted root vegetables for dinner and have some leftover, these can be combined with a grain, like brown rice, a bean, for example chickpeas, and some salad vegetables (like celery, radish, spinach), and you now have a filling lunchtime salad. Add a dressing and there you have it: filling, tasty and nutritious… and it hardly took more than 10 minutes to put together.

Make sure you buy some BPA-free containers, and avoid lunches that need to be microwaved. After all, heating food in a plastic container will only cause plastic to leach into your food. The chemicals in plastic are known to disrupt hormones, and that's the last thing you need when you're trying to heal PCOS.

This section is very short and contains only three recipes - don't let this alarm you, there are plenty more recipes in Chapter 5 which you can use for lunch as well. What I wanted to show you in this chapter is how simple it can be to create a salad for lunch. Think of this meal as an opportunity to give your body everything it needs to combat PCOS: a source of protein, complex carbohydrates, some healthy fats, and a good helping of vegetables.

POWER BOWLS

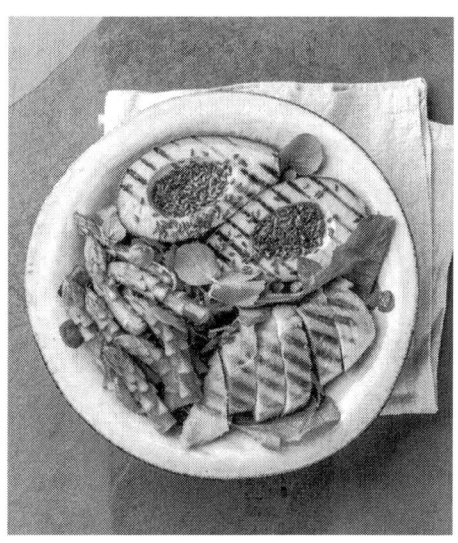

Power bowls are a fantastic way to make sure you get a good balance of nutrients in a convenient way. You can tailor your bowls to your own tastes and dietary requirements. They can be made in advance, stored in the fridge and taken to the office.

The kind of balance you want to aim for is:

- 1/4 of your plate filled with a grain (brown rice, wholegrain pasta, millet...)
- 1/4 of your plate filled with protein (aim for plant sources of protein; if you must have animal protein, buy organic & free-range poultry or meat, and wild-caught fish)

- 1/2 of your plate filled with vegetables (roasted vegetables, salad vegetables, salad leaves, etc.)
- A couple of tablespoons of dressing or a handful of toasted seeds, or a few cubes of vegan cheese (for added healthy fats, and because this will elevate your salad to gourmet status!).

Next, you'll find three of my favorite combinations, plus some ideas so you can start making your own.

TOFU AND AVOCADO POWER BOWL

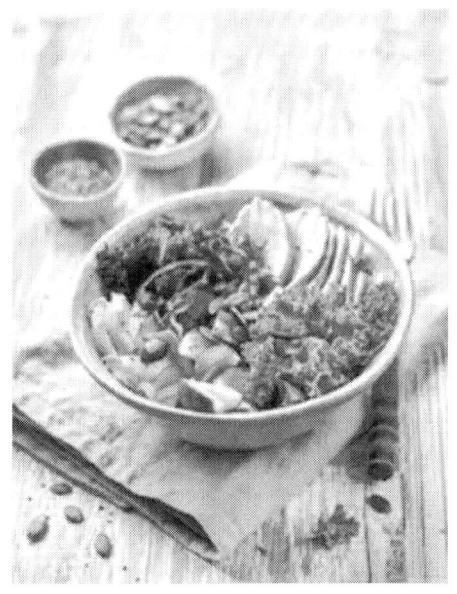

Ingredients (serves 1):

- 1 avocado (pitted and cut into pieces)
- 1/2 cup cooked quinoa
- 2 handfuls of baby spinach
- 1/2 cup smoked tofu (cut into small pieces)
- 1/2 lemon (juiced)
- 1 tbsp olive oil
- Pinch of salt
- 2 tbsp toasted almonds

Method:

1. The night before, cook the quinoa and allow to cool.

2. Bake the almonds in a pre-heated oven at 350F for 10-12 minutes. Allow to cool.

3. In your lunch container, layer the spinach, followed by the quinoa, avocado, and tofu. Sprinkle with the toasted almonds.

4. Seal, and keep in the fridge until you're ready to take it to work.

5. You can add the olive oil, lemon juice and salt in advance, or place these ingredients in a small pot to mix with the salad when you're ready to eat.

ROASTED VEG & CHICKPEA POWER BOWL

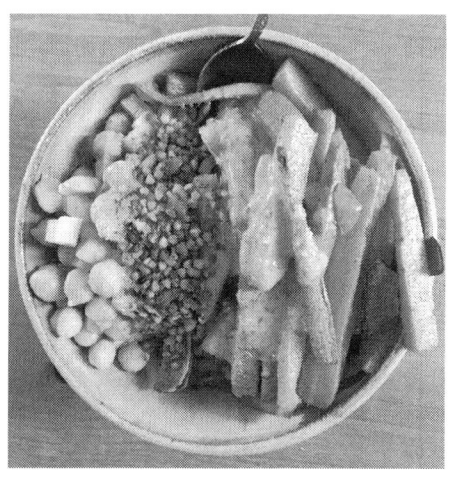

Ingredients (serves 1):

- 2 medium sweet potatoes
- 2 medium beetroots
- 2 medium carrots
- 1 tbsp coconut oil (melted)
- 2 tbsp mild curry powder
- 1/2 cup cooked chickpeas
- 1/2 cup cooked brown rice
- 2 celery sticks
- 1/2 lemon (juiced)
- Pinch of salt
- 2 tbsp cashew nuts (roughly chopped)

- 1 handful of baby spinach or other salad leaves

Method:

1. You can prepare the roasted vegetables the day before - there will be enough for a couple of meals.
2. Peel and chop the sweet potatoes, carrots and beetroot, taking care that the carrot and beetroot pieces are the same size, with the sweet potato pieces a little bigger.
3. In a large bowl, mix together the vegetable pieces with the melted coconut oil, curry powder, and a pinch of salt. Spread onto a baking tray lined with baking paper, and bake at 390F for 15-20 minutes. Allow to cool.
4. Chop the celery sticks into small pieces.
5. In a medium bowl, mix together the salad leaves, chickpeas, cooked brown rice, celery, cashew nuts, lemon juice and olive oil. Place the mix in your lunchbox.
6. Add about 1/2 cup of roasted vegetables. Close the box, refrigerate, and simply grab and go before work.

MEDITERRANEAN POWER BOWL

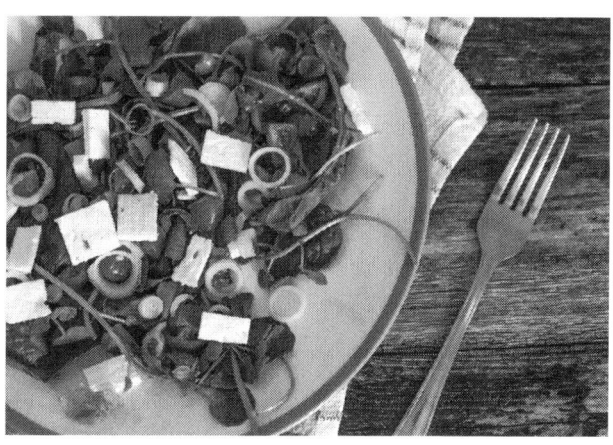

Ingredients (serves 1):

- 1/2 cup cooked millet
- 1/4 cup sweet pepper (finely sliced)
- 1/2 cup canned lentils (rinsed and drained)
- Handful of cherry tomatoes (chopped in half)
- Handful of arugula or watercress
- 1/4 cup cucumber (chopped into small pieces)
- 1/4 cup vegan feta cheese (chopped into cubes)
- 2 tbsp pine nuts
- 1/2 lemon (juiced)
- 1 tbsp olive oil
- Pinch of salt

- Small handful of fresh parsley (chopped finely)

Method:

1. Cook the millet the night before - you can batch cook enough for several meals and store extra portions in the fridge.
2. In a frying pan, toast the pine nuts for around 2 minutes, until they are lightly golden. Set aside.
3. In a large bowl, combine the cooked millet, sweet peppers, arugula, tomatoes, lentils, cucumber, lemon juice, olive oil, salt and parsley. Mix well.
4. Transfer into your lunchbox and top with vegan feta cheese and the toasted pine nuts. Keep chilled until it's time for lunch!

Handy Tip - How to Create Your Own Power Bowl

Variety is the spice of life! Power bowls make it easy to create tasty lunches that stay interesting throughout the week. Use these three versions as inspiration, and start making your own. Remember to balance protein, complex carbs, veggies, and a good source of healthy fats.

Keep things interesting by including different textures, and add a tasty dressing to marry it all together - you'll find three recipes for creamy salad dressings next.

Complex carbs (around a quarter of your plate):

- Quinoa
- Brown rice or black rice
- Buckwheat, buckwheat noodles or buckwheat pasta
- Brown rice pasta
- Millet

Protein and plant protein (around a quarter of your plate):

- Black beans, chickpeas, cannellini beans, kidney beans, mung beans, adzuki beans, lentils etc.
- Tofu or tempeh
- Vegan sausages
- Oily fish (salmon, mackerel, sardines, herring)
- Organic, free-range, humane egg, meat or poultry

Salad veggies (half your plate should be full of salad veggies or cooked veggies, or a combination of both):

- Kale / spinach / watercress / arugula / romaine lettuce / endive
- Cucumber
- Celery
- Radish
- Tomatoes

- Peppers
- Zucchini
- Carrots

Cooked veggies (half your plate should be full of salad veggies or cooked veggies, or a combination of both):

- Roasted root vegetables (beetroot, carrot, sweet potato, celeriac…)
- Steamed broccoli or cauliflower
- Grilled zucchini
- Grilled mushrooms

Healthy fats (top your lunch with a portion of healthy fats):

- Vegan cheese (1/4 cup)
- Avocado (1/2 or one)
- Nuts and seeds (1-3 tbsp)
- Olive oil (1 tbsp)

SALAD DRESSINGS

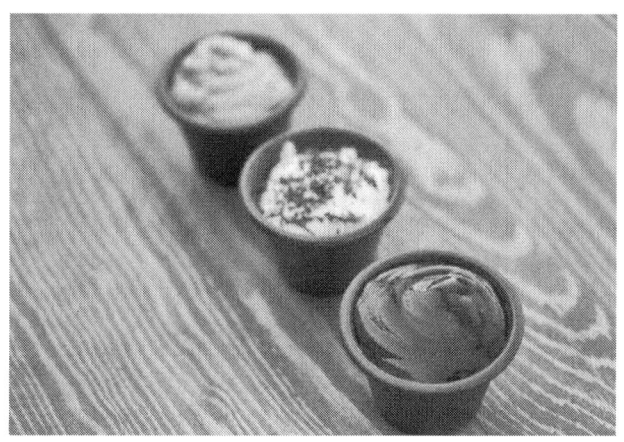

TURMERIC TAHINI DRESSING

Ingredients (makes around 1 cup):

- 3 tbsp tahini
- 3 tbsp olive oil
- 2/3 cup water (you may not need as much, depending how thick you like your dressings)
- 1 tsp turmeric powder
- Pinch of salt and pepper

Method:

1. In a medium bowl, mix together the tahini and olive oil until they are combined.
2. Add the turmeric and mix well.
3. Add the water a tablespoon or two at a time, mixing it into the tahini completely before adding more. Don't add all the water in one go otherwise the sauce will not emulsify.
4. Once you're happy with the consistency, season with salt and pepper.
5. Store in an airtight jar in the fridge for up to a week.

SPICY ALMOND DRESSING

Ingredients (makes around 1 cup):

- 3 tbsp almond butter
- 2/3 cup water (you may not need as much, depending how thick you like your dressings)
- 1-2 tsp mild curry powder
- Pinch of salt and pepper

Method:

1. In a medium bowl, mix together the almond butter and water - add a little water at a time, mixing until the butter is fully combined with the water before adding any more.
2. Once you're happy with the consistency, add the curry powder, salt and pepper and mix well. Taste and adjust seasoning if necessary.
3. Store in an airtight jar in the fridge for up to a week.

SMOKED PAPRIKA DRESSING

Ingredients (makes around 1 cup)

- 3 tbsp cashew nut butter
- 1/2 lemon (juiced)
- 2/3 cup water (you may not need as much, depending how thick you like your dressings)
- 1-2 tsp smoked paprika powder
- Pinch of salt

Method:

1. In a medium bowl, mix together the cashew butter and lemon juice until well combined.
2. Add a little water at a time, mixing until it is fully combined before adding any more.
3. Once you're happy with the consistency, add the smoked paprika powder, salt and pepper and mix well. Taste and adjust seasoning if necessary.
4. Store in an airtight jar in the fridge for up to a week.

CHAPTER FIVE:

MY FAVORITE DINNER RECIPES

Preparing a home-cooked meal and eating together around a table is, in our modern world, a bit of a luxury! For years, my husband and I relied on fast food and processed ready meals to satiate our hunger when we returned from a long day at work. The thought of slaving in the kitchen for hours to prepare a home-cooked meal was a completely alien concept, and honestly not one that I wanted to pursue. But I was wrong.

I can now officially say that it is far more enjoyable to come home after work and spend some time cooking together and sitting down to an enjoyable meal. We switch off the TV and we genuinely want to hear about each other's day.

The other thing I can say is that you don't have to slave over a hot stove for hours to prepare a tasty meal. In fact the recipes you'll find in this section are, for the most part, super speedy. You can always make a little extra and save it either for lunch the next day, or for dinner on a night you know you won't have the time or inclination to cook anything.

PUMPKIN AND SWEET POTATO SOUP

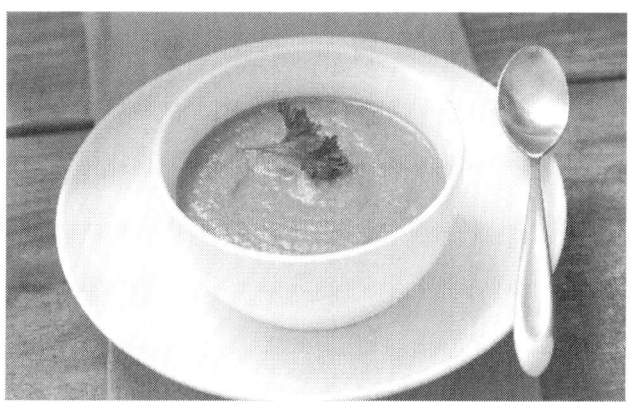

Soup is a great source of energy, and can be packed full of healthy protein and vegetables. Serve it with a slice of gluten-free whole grain bread, or a portion of high-protein grains like quinoa or buckwheat.

You can make enough soup for several meals. Once it is cooked, simply allow to cool, portion it out and refrigerate. Freeze any soup that will be eaten later than in three days' time. When you're ready, simply defrost for 24 hours in the fridge.

Ingredients (serves 4):

- 3 tbsp coconut oil
- 1 onion (finely diced)
- 2 cloves garlic (crushed)

88

- 4 cups vegetable stock
- 2 large sweet potato (peeled and diced)
- 1 small pumpkin or squash (peeled, seeds removed, and diced)
- 1/2 cup nutritional yeast or 1/2 cup coconut cream
- 1 tsp chili flakes (optional)

Method:

1. Heat the oil in a large saucepan and add the onion and garlic. Sauté until the onion is soft and the mixture is fragrant.
2. Add the vegetable stock, stir, and bring to the boil.
3. Add the chopped pumpkin and sweet potato, and simmer for 20-25 minutes, or until the sweet potato and pumpkin are soft.
4. Remove from the heat and allow to cool slightly, then use a hand blender to blend the mixture until smooth. If you don't have a hand blender, you can transfer to a blender or food processor in small amounts and then return back to the pot. Make sure you do NOT use a closed blender (like a Nutribullet) to blend soup, because the steam from the hot liquid can cause the blender to explode.
5. Return to the heat, stir in nutritional yeast or coconut cream, and add salt, pepper, and chili flakes to taste.

Handy Tips

Nutritional yeast is a great vegan seasoning to have in your kitchen cupboards. It has a mildly cheesy flavor, which can satisfy that craving for dairy. For example, you can mix it into pasta, sprinkle in on soups, or even blend it with soaked cashews to make a cheesy sauce.

MEXICAN STUFFED PEPPERS

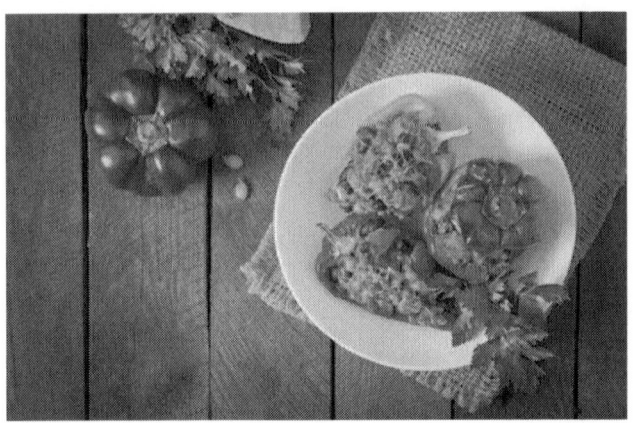

Perfect for dinner, fantastic as a leftover lunch, and great for entertaining. Any type of Mexican food can be instantly transformed into a feast, simply by adding a couple of healthy sides like homemade guacamole, hummus, or a black bean salad.

As you can see, eating healthy doesn't mean just eating lettuce. You can enjoy all types of food, just by making small adjustments - like swapping red meat for tofu or beans, or swapping white rice for whole grains, or simply by making sure there are enough vegetables on your plate.

Ingredients (makes 8 stuffed pepper halves):

- 4 large peppers (any color will do, or choose more than one color)

- 1 tbsp olive oil
- 1 cup black beans or adzuki beans (alternatively 1 cup ground organic grass-fed beef)
- 1 onion (finely diced)
- 1/2 cup tomato puree
- 1 tsp cumin powder
- 1 tsp chili powder
- 1/2 tsp salt
- 1/2 tsp cinnamon
- Vegan grated parmesan or vegan cheddar cheese

Method:

1. Cut the peppers vertically from the stem to base; remove all the seeds and core from the inside of the peppers.
2. Place the peppers hollow side up on a baking tray, cover with foil, and bake in a preheated oven at 350F for around 10-15 minutes.
3. While peppers are cooking, you can prepare the filling.
4. Heat the olive oil on medium, and sauté the onions until they are translucent.
5. Add the black beans or adzuki beans and the spices. Cook for a couple of minutes and then add the tomato purée. (If you are making this dish with beef, cook until the beef is browned and completely cooked).

6. Once the mixture is cooked, remove from the heat and spoon into the pepper shells.
7. Sprinkle with a vegan parmesan or cheddar cheese and then bake in the oven for around 10 minutes or until bubbly and golden.

Handy Tip

This is a beautiful recipe for entertaining - it looks great on a plate, is packed with flavor, and is relatively easy to make, even for large groups. You can also enjoy making this al fresco - grilling the peppers on the barbeque is another way to prepare them and will add a nice smoky flavor. Have fun with this recipe and freestyle:

- Fill the peppers with cooked brown rice, sautéed vegetables and north African spices instead.
- Replace the black beans with any other bean.
- Add finely sliced mushrooms or other vegetables to the bean mix.

AVOCADO WAFFLE TOAST

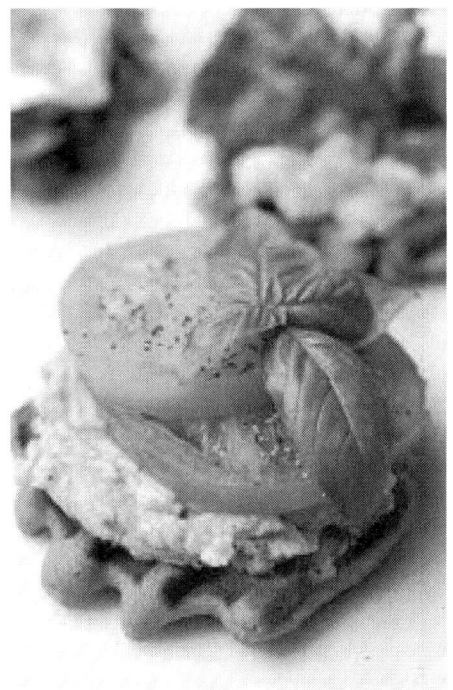

I know I know, waffles for dinner, really? But this is one to try when you fancy something a bit comforting and a bit different. It's a great one to have for brunch as well! You will need a waffle maker, but it's worth it!

Ingredients (serves 2):

- 1/2 cup almond butter
- 2 large organic free-range eggs

- 2 tbsp coconut oil (melted)
- ¼ cup almond milk
- 2 tbsp maple syrup
- 1/2 tsp Himalayan salt
- 1/2 tbsp baking soda
- 1/2 cup almond flour

For the topping, you will need:

- 2 avocados
- 1/2 lemon (juiced)
- 2 large tomatoes (sliced)
- A pinch of salt
- A pinch black pepper
- A few basil leaves

Method:

1. Preheat the waffle maker while you prepare your ingredients.
2. In a large bowl, whisk together the almond butter, eggs, melted coconut oil, almond milk, and maple syrup until well mixed together.
3. Add the almond flour, baking soda, and salt. Whisk to combine.
4. Oil the waffle grill to prevent sticking. Add 1/4 cup of batter and cook for about 5 minutes or until both sides are golden brown. Repeat for the remaining batter until it is all used up.
5. While the waffles are cooking, mash up the avocado in a bowl with a squeeze of lemon juice.

6. Spread mashed avocado on each waffle, top with a slice of tomato, a sprinkle of salt and pepper, and a basil leaf.

Handy Tips

There is something very comforting about a waffle - and these ones happen to be PCOS-friendly! As you can see, they're very easy to make. So why not make some different toppings? For example:

- Crunchy peanut butter with a sliced banana.
- Whipped coconut cream with strawberries.
- Hummus and sauerkraut.

LOW-CARB PASTA SAUCE

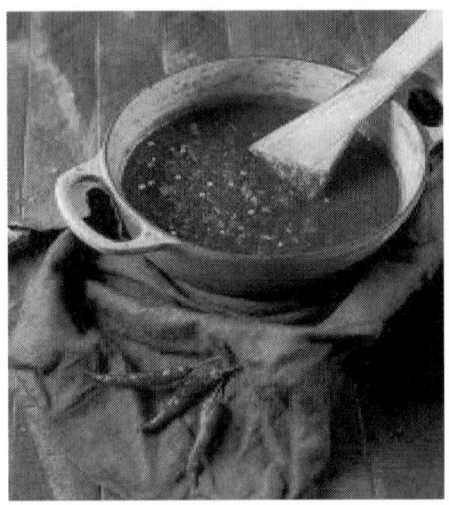

This delicious sauce takes under 10 minutes to make - perfect for pizza, but also a great base for vegetable pasta dishes like lasagna. What I love about homemade food is that it gives you the chance to tailor the flavor by adding spices and herbs of your choice.

Ingredients (serves 2-4)

For the basic sauce:

- 1 onion (finely sliced)
- 4 cloves garlic (minced)
- 2 tbsp olive oil
- 6 tbsp tomato paste

- 3 cups canned tomatoes (or 3 cups plum tomatoes, chopped)
- 2 tsp dried oregano
- 2 tsp dried parsley
- 1 tsp chili flakes
- 1/2 tsp salt
- 1/2 tsp black pepper

What you can add:

- 1 cup sliced mushrooms
- 1 zucchini (finely sliced)
- 1 can cannellini beans (rinsed and drained)
- 1 eggplant (chopped into small pieces)
- 1 leek (sliced finely)
- 2-3 sticks of celery (finely sliced)
- … or whatever vegetables you enjoy!

Method:

1. Heat the olive oil in a large saucepan and cook the onion and garlic until the onion is softening. Add the tomato paste and stir well.
2. Add the chopped tomatoes and herbs, stir, and leave to simmer for around 10 minutes.
3. If you are adding vegetables - add them with the chopped tomatoes and simmer gently for 10-20 minutes, or until the vegetables are cooked through.
4. Season with chili flakes, salt and black pepper.

Handy Tips

This sauce can be stored in a freezer and it will stay fresh for up to two months. It's a nice idea to make a large batch of the basic sauce and freeze it in portions. This way, if you get the urge to make a lasagna or some other vegetable pasta dish, you've got half the job done already.

VEGETABLE AND LENTIL SOUP

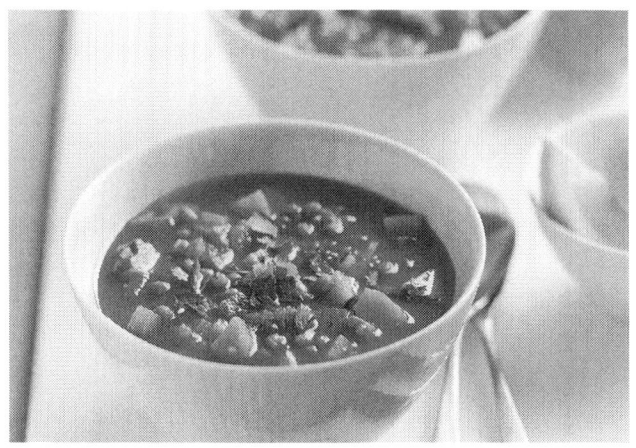

Ingredients (serves 4):

- 1 red onion (diced)
- 1 clove garlic (minced)
- 2 tbsp olive oil
- 1 cup dried lentils
- 4 cups vegetable stock
- 2 cans of chopped tomatoes
- 3 cups water
- 2 carrots (diced)
- 2 celery sticks (diced)
- 4 red potatoes (diced)
- A handful of fresh mint or parsley
- Pinch of salt and pepper

Method:

1. In a large saucepan, heat the olive oil. Add the onions, celery, and carrots.
2. Add the minced garlic and stir until the garlic begins to brown.
3. Add the lentils, vegetable stock, diced potatoes, water, and canned tomatoes. Stir to mix everything.
4. Bring to boil, then cover the pot and let it simmer for 45 minutes or until lentils are fully cooked.
5. Serve with a sprinkle of fresh parsley, and a side of grains.

Handy Tip

This dish can be served with a gluten-free bread, naan bread, or a portion of grains (think brown rice or quinoa). It can easily be frozen for another day.

You can create a completely different soup by using other ingredients:

- Use beans instead of lentils (but note that these will have to be pre-cooked).
- Try it with sweet potatoes and beetroot instead of carrots and potatoes.
- Add shredded cabbage or chopped kale.

ZOODLES WITH MEDITERRANEAN VEGETABLE SAUCE

Zoodle? What's one of those? Zoodles are noodles made from zucchini - but they can be made with carrots and cucumber too, and they are a healthy alternative to pasta since not only are they gluten-free, they maximize the amount of vegetables on your plate. I promise you will not miss pasta for a second.

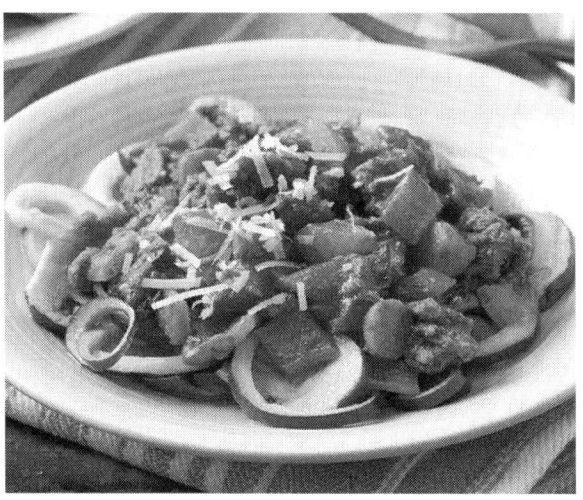

Ingredients (serves 2-4):
- 1/2 cup cooked kidney beans or 1/2 cup organic sustainable lean ground beef

- 1-2 medium carrots (chopped)
- 1 large onion (chopped)
- 3 sticks of celery (chopped)
- 1 cup mushrooms (sliced)
- 1 clove garlic (minced)
- 1 can chopped tomatoes
- 1 handful plum tomatoes (diced)
- 1/2 tsp Italian seasoning
- 1 cup zoodles (spiralized zucchini) - around 1-2 medium zucchini
- 2 tbsp vegan parmesan cheese or nutritional yeast

Method:

1. To make the sauce, heat the oil in a large saucepan, and cook the onion and garlic for a couple of minutes. Then add the beans, carrots, celery, and tomatoes. Cook until the vegetables are beginning to soften. Add the Italian seasoning.
2. If you are making this dish with meat, cook until the meat is tender.
3. Add the chopped tomatoes along with 1/2 cup of water, and stir. Bring to the boil and then simmer for 10-20 minutes. While that's cooking, boil a pot of lightly salted water for the zoodles.
4. Make the zoodles by spiralizing the zucchini.
5. Add the sliced mushrooms to the pasta sauce and cook for 2 more minutes.

6. Add the zoodles to the pot of boiling, salted water. Cook for 3 minutes. Drain the zoodles in a strainer.
7. To serve, top the zoodles with a big spoonful of pasta sauce. Sprinkle with parmesan or nutritional yeast.

Handy Tip:

- Try this dish with carrot noodles instead, they will add a pop of vibrant orange color to your dish.

BLACK BEAN BURGERS

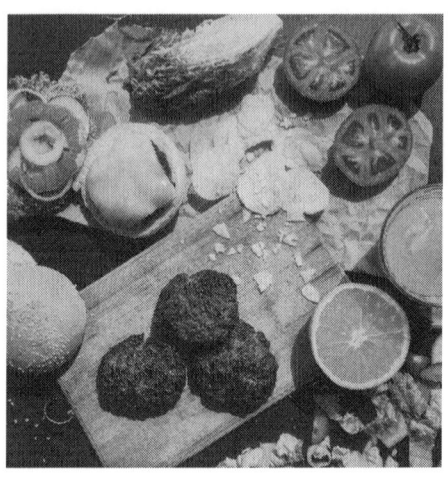

Ingredients (makes 4 burgers):

- 1 cup walnuts
- 1 onion (chopped)
- 1 clove garlic (crushed)
- 1 tbsp olive oil
- 1 can of black beans (drained)
- 1 tsp smoked paprika
- 1 tsp cumin
- 2 tbsp tomato paste
- 1 tsp salt
- 1/2 cup oat flour (plus a bit more if needed)
- 2 tbsp olive oil (for frying)

Method:

1. Place the walnuts in a food processor, and process until they're a medium crumb. Set aside.
2. Place the olive oil in a frying pan; fry the onion and crushed garlic until the onions are soft. Take care not to burn the garlic.
3. Transfer the fried onions to a food processor along with the black beans, paprika, cumin, tomato paste and salt. Process until combined.
4. In a large bowl, place the bean mix, the walnut crumb and the oat flour, and mix. If your mix is very wet, add a little more flour.
5. Divide your mix into four, roll it into balls and press onto a tray lined with baking paper. Pat them into burger patty shapes.
6. Place in the freezer for 30 minutes to firm up. This will help them hold together when you fry them.
7. Add 2 tbsp olive oil to a frying pan, and fry the burgers for 5 minutes on each side.
8. Serve with your choice of salad, or in a gluten-free bun with some baby spinach and sliced tomatoes.

Handy Tip:

My go-to dish when I fancy something traditional, without the red meat. You can play around with this recipe by using different beans - chickpeas work very well - and swapping the spices. For example, using curry spices instead of paprika and cumin, or using ground almonds instead of walnuts.

GRILLED SALMON WITH BASIL

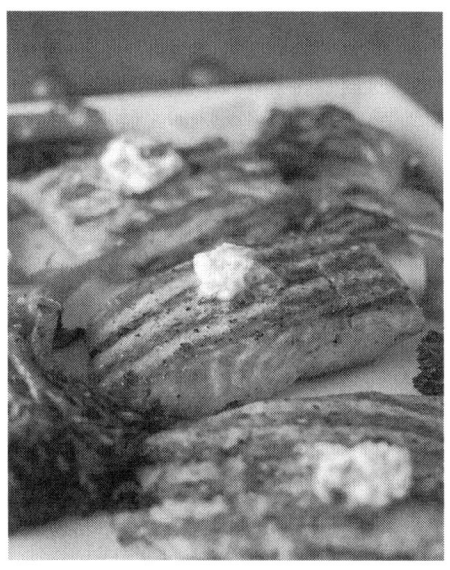

Ingredients (serves 4):

- 4 salmon steaks
- 2 tbsp lemon juice
- 2 tbsp avocado oil
- 1 tbsp dried and crushed basil
- 4 lemon wedges

Method:

1. In a small bowl, mix together the lemon juice, basil, and avocado oil.
2. Place the salmon steaks on a tray lined with

baking paper; brush the mixture on, making sure the salmon is completely coated.

3. Grill the salmon on medium heat for about ten minutes (for every inch of thickness). Or grill until the salmon flakes when you test it with a fork. Check the salmon is cooked before serving: the internal temperature should be around 145F.

4. Serve the salmon with lemon wedges.

Handy Tips

Oily fish like salmon can be a good source of healthy fats and Omega-3 fatty acids. You can serve these salmon steaks alongside a fresh salad or half an avocado - the perfect light dinner! You can also substitute the salmon for other oil fish like herring or mackerel.

KETO PALEO SHRIMP AND MINCED CHICKEN SHUMAI

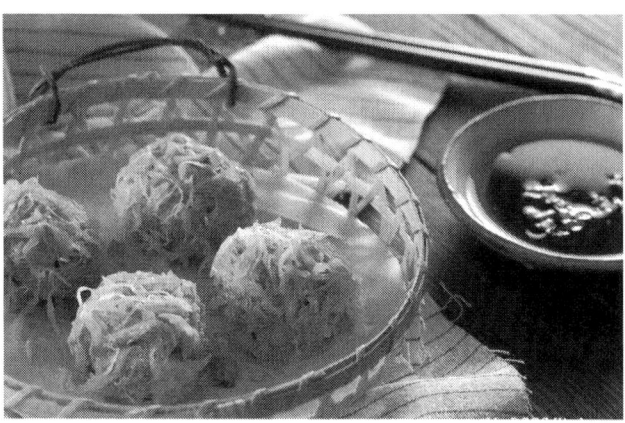

It might look complicated, but this is a very quick and simple dish that, once you've had it, will become a firm favorite. This recipe is a Chinese-restaurant inspired dim sum dish that is sure to impress your friends and family. You can also keep the leftovers for your lunch the next day.

Ingredients (serves 4):

- 1 large cabbage
- 3 cups minced chicken (organic, free-range)
- 3 cups peeled shrimp (sustainably sourced)
- OR - sub the chicken and shrimp with a soy-based meat alternative
- 1 green onion/scallion (chopped)

- 1/2 red onion (minced)
- 1 tbsp ginger (minced)
- 2 tbsp coconut aminos
- 2 tbsp sesame oil
- 1/2 tbsp pink salt
- 1/2 tbsp black pepper

For the dipping sauce:

- 2 tbsp coconut aminos
- 1 tbsp white vinegar
- 1 tbsp chili oil
- 1 tbsp sesame oil

Method:

1. Chop the shrimp and chicken (or soy chunks) into small pieces.
2. Mince the red onion and the green onion together.
3. In a large bowl, mix together the onions, chicken, shrimp, ginger, coconut aminos, sesame oil, salt and pepper, until well combined.
4. Using your hands, roll meatballs of your desired size.
5. Using a shredder or a sharp knife, shred the cabbage very finely.
6. Roll each meatball in the shredded cabbage until they are well coated.
7. Place the coated meatballs on parchment paper, and place this in a vegetable steamer to steam

for around 15 minutes. Alternatively, heat 1 cup of water in a wok and use a bamboo steamer.
8. While the shumai are cooking, mix the dipping sauce ingredients in a bowl.
9. Serve hot and enjoy with the dipping sauce.

Handy Tip

You can veganize this dish by using Quorn or another plant-based meat alternative instead of the chicken and shrimp.

ROASTED BROCCOLI
WITH BASIL SAUCE

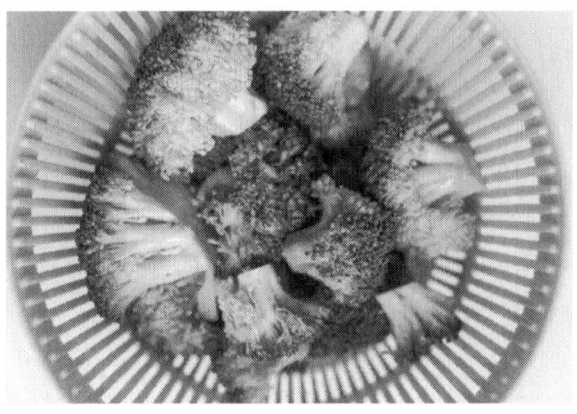

The best way to eat more greens is to make them irresistible with the addition of a dressing or plenty of seasoning. This dish roasts broccoli to give it a delicious smoky flavor, then tops it with a cooling and creamy basil sauce. Broccoli has never tasted so good.

Ingredients (serves 2):

- 1 large broccoli (cut into florets)
- 2 tsp coconut oil (melted)
- Pinch of pink salt
- Pinch garlic powder
- Pinch of cayenne pepper (optional - leave out if you don't like spicy food)

For the basil sauce:

- 1/2 cup cashew nuts (soaked for 4 hours and drained)
- 1/2 cup plant milk (almond milk or soy milk work well)
- A small handful of fresh basil
- 2 tbsp nutritional yeast
- 1 tbsp olive oil
- Pinch pink salt

Method:

1. Preheat the oven to 400F.
2. In a medium bowl, place the broccoli florets, the garlic powder, salt, coconut oil and cayenne pepper. Mix until everything is evenly distributed.
3. Spread the broccoli florets on a baking tray and bake for 15-20 minutes, depending on the size of the florets.
4. While the broccoli is roasting, make the basil dressing.
5. Place the soaked cashew nuts, plant milk, basil, nutritional yeast, olive oil and pink salt in a high-speed blender, and blend until completely smooth.
6. Drizzle the basil sauce over the roasted broccoli and serve.

Handy Tip

This recipe also tastes great cold - it can be part of one of your power bowls! You can double up the basil sauce and store the leftovers in the fridge. It works well with other vegetables, as a creamy salad dressing, and even stirred into pasta.

You can freestyle this dish:

- Use cauliflower instead of broccoli.
- Swap the fresh basil for a piece of fresh turmeric root and a pinch of curry spices.
- Swap the basil for lemon juice and the sauce will be more like mayonnaise!
- Use the sauce as a dip for raw vegetables - perfect party food!

Some of the dinner recipes I have shared with you may take a little more prep time than you may be willing to set aside for now. If that is the case, don't panic - just focus on the shorter recipes in this book, and use them to create quick healthy dinners. There's nothing stopping you, for example, having a power bowl for dinner! But, if you can, just one night a week, give yourself the gift of spending some time leisurely making yourself dinner. Cooking doesn't have to be stressful - in fact, it is a beautiful act of self-care.

In the next chapter, I'll share my favorite veggie and vegan recipes, followed by the chapter we've all been waiting for… healthy treats and desserts!

CHAPTER SIX:

MY FAVORITE VEGAN AND VEGETARIAN RECIPES

I wrote these recipes with non-vegans in mind, because I believe that in order for a recipe to be great, everyone should be able to enjoy it.

There are different schools of thought when it comes to the benefits of eating meat for PCOS. Plenty of people have gone on keto diets (where carbs are kept to a strict minimum, while animal protein is abundant) and have found their PCOS symptoms improve. But this is not to do with the meat, it is to do with reducing carbs and generally eating "cleaner" - in other words, swapping processed foods for home cooked foods.

In fact, there is an overwhelming body of evidence showing that a plant-based diet benefits your entire health, not just your hormones - it reduces the risk of chronic disease and improves longevity. In this chapter, I want to share a few more recipes - not to bully you into going vegan, but rather to show you that you can easily include more plant-based dishes into your day, and that it doesn't necessarily have to mean eating only lentils and cabbage.

It is ok if you don't feel ready to go totally vegan. The important thing is that you begin to reduce your meat consumption - bit by bit, a little more every week. It is easy to give up dairy, because there are now so many plant alternatives for milk, cream, and even cheese. Meat, on the other hand, can be a little bit tricky - but once you've made a few vegan dishes, you'll find it much easier to think of your meals in terms of overall ingredients rather than just "meat and sides." What's more, when you experience just how tasty and filling vegan food can be, you'll feel more comfortable with including more plants in your life. Don't put pressure on yourself, just give it a try, keep an open mind, and experience the benefits for yourself.

ASPARAGUS RISOTTO

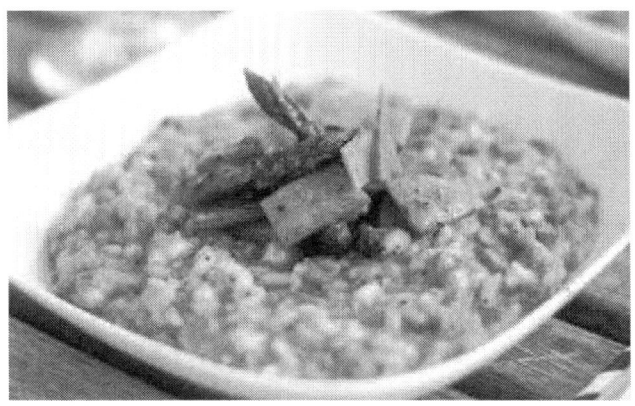

Asparagus is a great source of prebiotic fiber - fiber that feeds your good bacteria. So it's well worth adding it to your diet. Risotto is one of my favorite dishes, especially when I have guests coming over... and the best thing? While traditional risotto contains a lot of butter and cheese, vegan risotto is packed with plant goodness. You can also make it in bulk and freeze for future dinners and lunches.

Ingredients (serves 6):

- 2 cups of asparagus (with the ends cut off and chopped into 1-inch segments)
- 8 cups of vegetable stock
- 1 tbsp olive oil
- 1 handful scallions (chopped)

- 2 cups of short-grain brown rice
- 1 tbsp fresh lemon juice
- 3 tbsp nutritional yeast
- Salt and pepper

Method:

1. Steam the asparagus for around 5 minutes, or until it is cooked.
2. While the asparagus is steaming, bring the vegetable broth to the boil.
3. In a separate pan, heat the olive oil and sauté the scallions until they begin softening.
4. Add the brown rice and cook the mixture on medium heat, stirring continuously, for around 2-3 minutes.
5. Add the lemon juice and around 2-3 cups of the vegetable stock, mix well.
6. Add the rest of the stock gradually, around 1/2 cup at a time, mixing as you go, until the mixture absorbs the broth.
7. It will take around 40-45 minutes to cook the risotto. Make sure you stir the rice constantly as this will develop the starch that creates that creamy consistency you are looking for.
8. Once the rice is cooked through and all the liquid is evaporated, you can add the asparagus.
9. Add the nutritional yeast, salt, and pepper to taste, mix well, and serve.

Handy Tips

Risotto is best served family-style, with a huge bowl in the middle of the table and fresh salad. It also makes a great addition to barbeques and outdoor eating in the summer. It is essentially a rice dish, so watch your portion size with this one. You can keep it PCOS-friendly by pairing it with a big salad and a portion of protein, for example a bean burger or salmon.

ZUCCHINI LASAGNA

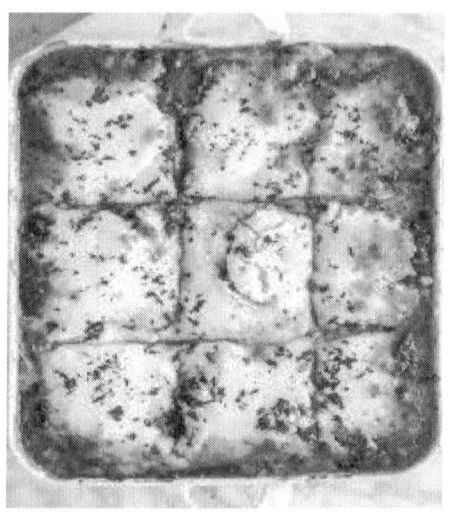

When I was first researching recipes for my new gluten free vegan diet, zucchinis were something I really struggled to cook with. However, I eventually learned to love it - I'm not sure why I didn't before! Zucchinis are a flexible and versatile vegetable that can be used as a replacement for carb-heavy pasta - for example in lasagna, or as noodles.

It's a good idea to note that zucchini contains a lot of water. You don't have to worry about this so much when making zoodles, but for this lasagna dish, you'll need to pre-cook it to avoid ending up with a really soggy dish.

This lasagna is an excellent crowd pleaser, for vegans and meat-eaters alike. The macadamias create a deliciously creamy and decadent béchamel layer that will satisfy even the most demanding diner.

Ingredients (serves 6-8):

- 2 cups macadamia nuts or cashew nuts (soaked for at least 4 hours, and drained)
- 4 medium zucchini squash (sliced and pre-grilled)
- 1 cup water (you might not use it all, but have on standby)
- 2 tbsp nutritional yeast
- 2/3 cup fresh basil (finely chopped)
- 1 1/2 tsp fresh oregano
- 1/2 a lemon (juiced)
- 1 tbsp olive oil
- Salt and pepper to taste
- 2-3 cups of tomato sauce (see recipe in Chapter 5)

Method:

1. Grill the zucchini under a medium heat for around 5 minutes on either side. Set aside.
2. Preheat the oven heated to 375F.
3. Blend the macadamia nuts (or cashew nuts) in a high-speed blender until they become a smooth

mixture - you may need to add a little bit of water to achieve this.

4. Then, add the nutritional yeast, olive oil, basil, oregano, lemon juice, salt and pepper, and blend until completely smooth.

5. Spoon a layer of tomato sauce onto the base of your oven dish.

6. Place the grilled zucchini slices on top of the sauce, and then top the zucchini with a quarter of the macadamia sauce.

7. Repeat this, creating layers of zucchini, tomato sauce and macadamia béchamel, finishing with a top layer of both sauces. Sprinkle with a little more nutritional yeast.

8. Cover with foil and bake in the oven for around 45 minutes.

9. Remove the foil and bake for a further 10 minutes.

10. Serve alongside a fresh salad.

Handy Tips

The perfect dish for guests since you can make a larger amount quite easily to accommodate more people. Don't be scared to try out other "pasta" layers - for example, you could grill slices of eggplant - which would turn this lasagna into a bit of a moussaka. Or you could use gluten-free pasta sheets made of lentils or chickpeas to add a source of protein.

The whole point of this new lifestyle is to try new things. The more cooking you do, the less afraid you will be of it. The beauty of vegan cooking is it can't really go wrong - as long as you choose vegetables you enjoy, chances are the result will be tasty.

You can have a lot of fun with cooking, and experimenting is a great way to introduce children or fussy eaters to plant-based meals, particularly if you make spiralized zucchini or cucumber! What's more, if you get your family involved you don't have to go through this alone and it will be so much easier to stick to your new healthy diet.

PORTOBELLO ROAD BURGER

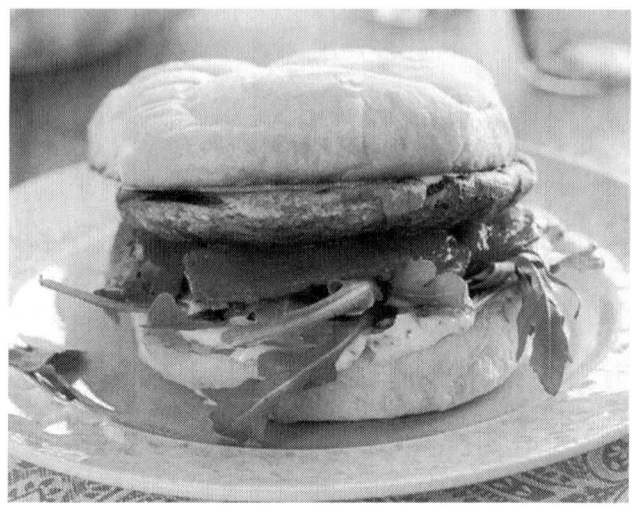

I was lucky enough to visit the world-famous Portobello Road during a recent trip to London. This recipe was named after that visit: the Portobello Road Burger!

Portobello mushrooms have long been a vegan staple and typical replacement for a juicy beef steak. Even though meat alternatives are getting fancier and more realistic all the time, there's a special place in my heart for mushrooms. They make for a tasty alternative, especially when you add the right seasonings.

Ingredients (serves 2-4):

- 4 Portobello mushrooms
- 1 tbsp olive oil
- 1 large onion (finely chopped)
- 1 handful of parsley (finely chopped)
- 2-3 celery stalks (finely chopped)
- 1 clove garlic (crushed)
- 1 tsp fresh thyme (finely chopped)
- 1 tsp oregano (finely chopped)
- 1/2 tsp sage (finely chopped)
- 1 tbsp tamari or soy sauce
- 1 tsp salt
- 2 cups gluten-free bread crumbs
- Gluten-free burger buns or other bun alternatives

Method:

1. Process the mushrooms and parsley in a food processor until fully mixed; set the mixture aside.
2. In a frying pan, heat the olive oil and sauté the garlic and onions until they start to brown.
3. Add the celery and sauté for another minute.
4. Transfer the sautéed vegetables to the bowl containing the mushroom and parsley mixture.
5. Add the thyme, oregano, sage, tamari sauce and breadcrumbs and mix well using a wooden spoon or your hands.

6. Place the mixture in the fridge for around one hour.
7. Once the mixture has cooled, preheat your oven to 350F.
8. Remove the mixture from the refrigerator.
9. With your hands, shape the mix into patties and place on a parchment-lined baking tray. For this part, you might want to wet your hands slightly, as it helps with the shaping process and keeping the mixture together.
10. Once all the patties are formed, place the tray in the oven for 20-30 minutes, checking occasionally to ensure they are cooked through.
11. You can then serve these on gluten-free rolls, or alongside some grains and veggies in your power box.

Handy Tips

For a burger with even fewer carbs, you can replace the bun with crisp fresh lettuce leaves and you'll enjoy maximum taste while avoiding that "too full to move" feeling... although, given that this is a mushroom burger, that's quite unlikely!

Burgers are a real treat, especially now that there are so many "realistic" plant-based alternatives on the market. However, these shop-bought alternatives aren't always very healthy. By playing around with this recipe and adjusting your seasonings as you go, you can create a tasty, low-calorie, meat-free alternative that you can easily make at home.

Another great way to use Portobello mushrooms in a burger is to use the mushroom caps as a burger "bun". Then for the "meat", you can choose from any number of delicious and nutritious vegan alternatives - a bean burger, tofu, or even soy meat. Simply grill the caps and voila - you've got yourself a quirky alternative to the standard burger bun.

PUMPKIN AND KALE SALAD

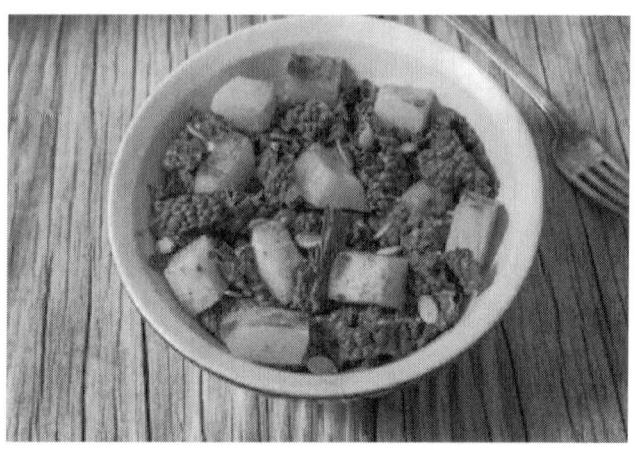

Kale is a wonderful superfood in the battle against PCOS, because it is low in carbohydrates but packed with antioxidants. Pumpkin makes a good addition thanks to its high fiber content, which helps slow the release of sugars and improve insulin sensitivity. Combine the two and you've got yourself a salad that tackles PCOS from all angles... and it just happens that it's also delicious!

Ingredients (serves 2):

- One bunch of kale (de-stemmed and chopped)
- 1/2 a red onion (sliced)
- 1/2 a pumpkin (peeled, deseeded, and sliced)
- 1 handful of hazelnuts

- 1 handful pomegranate seeds
- 1 tbsp olive oil
- 1/2 lemon (juiced)
- 1/2 tsp salt
- 1/2 tsp black pepper
- Healthy dressing of your choice (see dressing recipes in Chapter 4)

Method:

1. Preheat the oven to 375F.
2. Place the pumpkin slices and onion on a baking tray with parchment paper. Sprinkle with salt and pepper, and drizzle with olive oil.
3. Roast for about 20 minutes. Allow to cool completely.
4. While the vegetables are roasting, remove the stem from the kale, and roughly chop the leaves. Place them in a bowl with a sprinkle of salt and a little lemon juice and massage it. This will cause the kale to soften, and make it more pleasant to eat.
5. Add the roasted pumpkin, onion, pomegranate seeds and hazelnuts to the kale. Mix well.
6. Drizzle with a dressing of your choice and serve alongside bean burgers.

Handy Tips

The key thing to remember with salads is to use a dressing. A good dressing will turn those vegetables from boring to out of this world. Head back to the Power Bowls section and choose a dressing to add to this dish. My personal favorite is the smoked paprika dressing.

LOW-CARB NAAN-STYLE BREAD

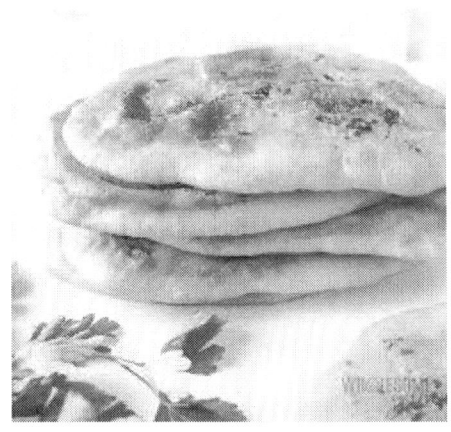

This Indian-style flatbread is a healthy alternative to regular naan bread. It is easy to make and dairy-free if you choose a vegan cheese for my cheese-stuffed option below, making it an excellent PCOS-diet addition. You can enjoy this naan bread with soup, or you can make pair it with a spicy curry.

Ingredients (serves 2-4):

Dry ingredients:

- 1/2 cup coconut flour
- 1 cup blanched almond flour
- 3 tablespoons powdered psyllium husk
- 1 tablespoon baking powder
- 1 tablespoon powdered onion

- 1 tablespoon powdered garlic
- 1 tablespoon curry powder
- 1/2 tablespoon salt

Wet ingredients:

- 3 eggs
- 1 cup hot water

Topping:

- 3 garlic cloves (minced)
- 1 tbsp olive or avocado oil

For cheese-stuffed bread:

- 2 cups vegan shredded mozzarella cheese

Method:

1. Preheat your oven to 375F.
2. In a large bowl, mix the dry ingredients.
3. Add the eggs and mix with a spatula well combined.
4. Add 1/4 cup of hot water to the batter and mix. Continue adding water in small amounts until you cannot mix the dough with the spatula.
5. Knead the dough with your hands until it forms a big, even-toned ball.
6. Separate the dough into medium-sized balls.
7. At this stage, you can choose to make plain naan bread or vegan cheese-stuffed bread.

Plain naan bread:

1. Place a dough ball on a piece of parchment paper and cover with another piece of parchment paper.
2. Roll the balls one at a time with a rolling pin until ¼-½ cm thick.
3. Transfer to a baking tray, removing the top layer of parchment paper.
4. Brush olive oil over the bread and sprinkle with minced garlic.
5. Place in the oven and bake for a maximum of 20 minutes, flip half way through, and keep your eye on them so they don't burn.
6. Serve hot.

Vegan cheese-stuffed bread:

1. Repeat the above method for rolling out the dough until all dough balls have been rolled out flat.
2. After you have rolled out all the dough, sprinkle 1/4 cup vegan cheese on half of your breads, then cover with a plain rolled dough.
3. Cover the dough with parchment paper and roll it out again so that the two are stuck together.
4. Transfer to a baking tray.
5. Brush with olive oil and sprinkle with minced garlic.
6. Bake for a maximum of 20 minutes, flip half way

through, and keep your eye on them to make
sure they don't burn.

7. Serve hot.

Handy Tips

Make sure that you use ground psyllium husk
and no other alternative. Since there is no gluten in
this recipe, it's the psyllium husk that will bind
everything together. When you add the hot water,
the psyllium husk will combine with the coconut
flour, expanding and stretching well.

You can swap the spices for other spices or herbs
of your choice. For example, you could use Italian
seasoning and turn these naan breads into
Mediterranean style breads instead.

ROASTED CAULIFLOWER & QUINOA SALAD

This hearty salad combines protein from the quinoa and complex carbs from the cauliflower, for a lunch that will keep you satisfied and energized for hours. A great dish to make in advance. It works well as an accompaniment to bean burgers.

Ingredients (serves 2):

- 1 large cauliflower
- 1 tbsp coconut oil (melted)
- 1 tbsp mild curry spice
- 1/2 tsp pink salt
- 1 handful baby spinach
- 1 cup cooked quinoa
- 2 dried apricots, chopped into small pieces OR 2 tbsp sultanas
- Juice and zest of 1 lime

Method:

1. Break up the cauliflower into small florets.
2. In a bowl, toss the florets in the coconut oil, curry spices and salt until evenly coated.
3. Place onto an oven tray lined with baking paper and bake for 15-20 minutes at 380F.

4. Wash and shred the spinach leaves.
5. Once the cauliflower is cooked, place it into a bowl with the quinoa, spinach, apricots, lime juice and lime zest, and mix well.
6. Serve warm, or allow to cool and store in an airtight container in the fridge. Keeps for 3 days.

SIMPLE SAUERKRAUT

Fermented foods are packed with good bacteria that replenish your gut flora. Sauerkraut is easy to make, and will add a zing to all your meals. Simply spoon it on top of salads, add it to wraps, or pile it onto oat crackers with hummus. Delicious and gut-friendly!

Ingredients (makes a 1-quart jar):

- 1 large cabbage (red or white)
- 2 tbsp Himalayan salt
- 1/2 - 1 cup raw apple cider vinegar
- 1/2 tbsp mustard seeds or 1/2 tbsp fennel seeds

Method:

1. Finely shred the cabbage.
2. Place it in a large pot, and sprinkle with salt. Mix and leave for 30 minutes.
3. With clean hands, massage the cabbage until it begins to soften and release its juices.
4. If adding mustard seeds or fennel seeds, add them to the cabbage once it softened.
5. Place the cabbage in a sterilized jar. Push the cabbage down so that it releases the juices. Add

the apple cider vinegar so that all the cabbage is submerged in liquid.

6. Close the jar and leave it on your kitchen worktop for 5 days, then move to the fridge, where it will keep fermenting. Open the jar every couple of days to allow the gases to escape.

7. You can eat it after 5 days, but it is better if you can leave it for 2 weeks until all the good bacteria to develop.

CHAPTER SEVEN:

DESSERTS AND TREATS

No diet can be complete without a few treats. And I'm happy to say that even on your new healthy lifestyle, you can enjoy the occasional dessert. That's right, treats don't have to be packed with sugar - and if they're not packed with sugar, they're safe to include in your PCOS-friendly diet.

Your new lifestyle isn't about being miserable or feeling like you can't enjoy in all life has to offer. By making some small changes, you can actually enjoy life much more and have the health, fitness, and energy to make the most of it.

AVOCADO MARGARITA

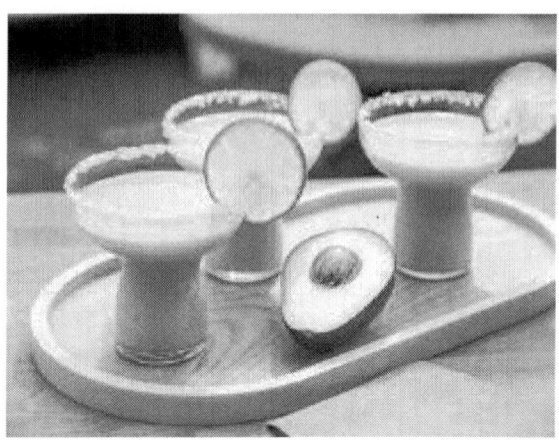

Margaritas were one of my absolute favorite drinks before I gave up alcohol, so imagine my delight when I realized there was a PCOS-friendly version I could enjoy. I did tell you that avocados were a superfood, but I bet you never thought we would have them in a margarita!

Ingredients (serves 2):

- 1 avocado (stone and skin removed)
- 3/4 cup lime juice
- 1 tsp maple syrup
- 1/2 cup orange juice
- 1/2 cup crushed ice
- 2 tsp salt
- 1 lime wedge

Method:

1. Pour the salt into a saucer.
2. Rub the edge of two martini glasses with the lime wedge and then place the rim in the salt, lining it with a light dusting of salt.
3. Blend the avocado, lime juice, orange juice, maple syrup, and ice in a blender.
4. Pour into margarita glasses and garnish with a slice of fresh lime.

Handy Tips

If you want to make this drink with alcohol, you of course absolutely can… but wherever possible, try and enjoy the virgin version as it's healthier and there is no disappointing hangover!

VANILLA BLUEBERRY CHEESECAKE MINI BITES

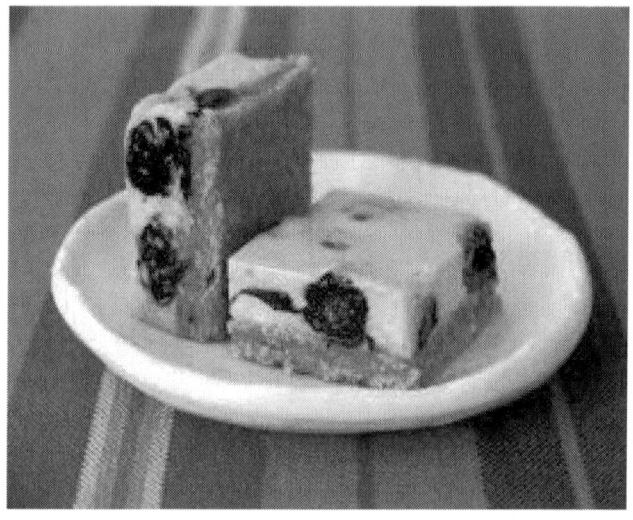

Who doesn't love cheesecake for dessert? Well, you'll be happy to find out you can make a healthy, PCOS-friendly version from scratch, that tastes just as good as the real thing!

For this recipe, I have made cheesecake mini bites, so you'll have portions you can either keep as a handy snack or for guests. However, this recipe will work just as well if you want to use a round cake tin. Just be careful you leave it to chill for long enough.

Ingredients (makes 10-12 bites):

For the crust:

- 1 cup almond meal
- 2 tbsp maple syrup
- 1 tbsp coconut oil (melted)
- 1 tsp vanilla extract
- 1/2 tsp salt

For the filling:

- 1 1/2 cups cashews (soaked overnight, rinsed and drained)
- 3 tbsp maple syrup
- 1 tsp vanilla extract
- 1/2 tsp salt
- 1/4 cup liquid coconut oil
- 2 vanilla beans (scraped from pod)
- 2 tbsp water

For the compote:

- 2 cups fresh blueberries
- 1/2 cup water
- 1/2 cup xylitol
- 2 tbsp lemon juice
- 2 tbsp cornstarch mixed with 2 tbsp water
- 1/2 tsp vanilla extract
- Zest of 1 lemon

Method:

For the crust:

1. Combine all ingredients in a food processor until it forms a crumbly mixture.
2. Spoon even amounts in mini cupcake molds, allowing for about 1 inch of crust for each cheesecake.
3. Press the mixture down into the cupcake containers.

For the filling:

1. Place all the ingredients in a blender and blend until completely smooth.
2. Pour into each of the cupcake molds; make sure you leave some room for your blueberry compote to go on the top.
3. Place in the freezer to set.

For the compote:

1. Combine blueberries, water, xylitol, and lemon juice in a pan and bring to a boil while stirring continuously.
2. Whisk cornstarch together with 2 tbsp of cold water and add to the blueberry mix. Allow to simmer until the sauce thickens, stirring constantly.
3. Once the mixture starts to thicken, remove from the heat and stir in the lemon zest.

4. Transfer to a bowl, and allow to cool.
5. Remove the mini cheesecakes from the freezer, add a spoonful of blueberry compote to each, and then return to the freezer to set for around 2 hours.

Handy Tips

You can replace blueberries with other berries, like cherries, strawberries or raspberries. The great thing about a recipe like this is that the cheesecake will last in your freezer for months, so you'll have a handy dessert you can serve at any time. Your friends won't believe it's vegan and healthy!

LEMON BAR FAT BOMBS

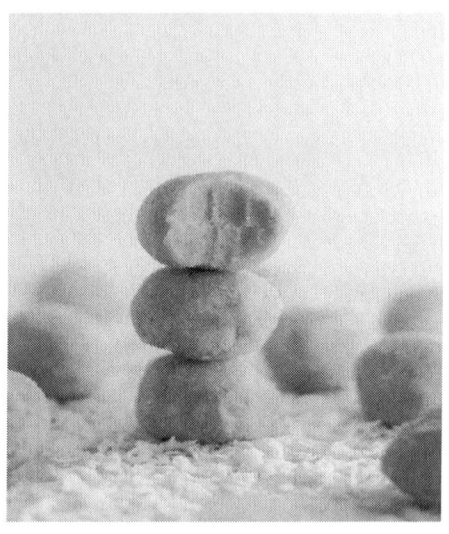

Healthy fat tastes good, feeds your brain, and keeps you full. These lemon bars will energize you for hours. I refer to them as my little power-packed balls of joy. And what is more impressive is that you can make them in bulk, store them in the freezer, and grab one anytime you feel hungry or when your cravings hit. These are a delicious vegan treat with a low carb content. They're also dairy-free and refined-sugar-free.

Ingredients (makes around 16-20 balls):

- 2 cups raw cashews (soaked overnight, rinsed and drained)

147

- 1/2 cup coconut butter
- 1 cup melted coconut oil
- 1 large lemon (zested)
- 1 cup lemon juice
- 1/4 cup coconut flour
- 1/2 cup shredded coconut
- Pinch salt
- 1/8 teaspoon stevia powder

Method:

1. Place all the ingredients in a food processor. Process until evenly mixed.
2. Transfer to a medium bowl and place in the fridge for up to 30 minutes - this will firm up the mixture enough for you to roll. (Alternatively, you can pour this mixture into a lined container and simply cut it into squares once it is set.)
3. Remove the bowl from the freezer and start rolling the mixture into small balls.
4. Place the balls on a baking sheet and put them back in the freezer for another 20 minutes.
5. Once hardened, transfer to an airtight container. You can either keep them in the freezer, where they will last for months, or in the fridge, where they will last around a week.

Handy Tips

Allow the balls to thaw for a few minutes if you're eating them straight from the freezer.

Be careful how much stevia you use, as the strength will depend on the brand. Some brands are more potent than others, and a little goes a long way. Taste the mixture before you start rolling, to make sure the balance is right for you.

NO-BAKE GRASSHOPPER BARS

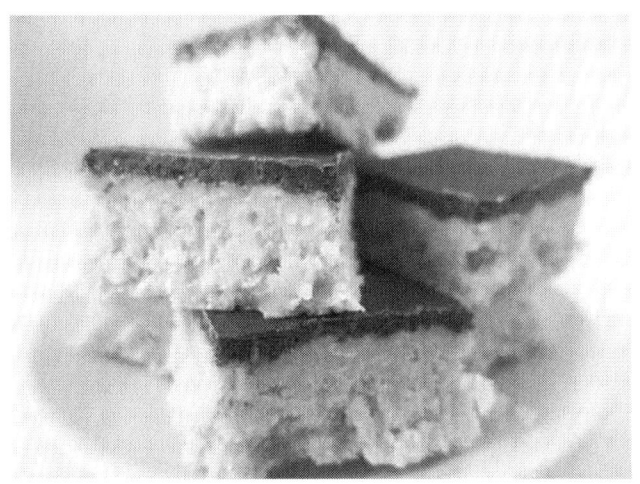

These bars are low in carbs and the perfect pick-me-up for when you fancy something sweet. They have two layers - a rich, coconutty-mint layer, topped with a decadent chocolate layer - perfect for when you need to curb those cravings. Full of healthy fat from avocados and coconut, your friends will be begging for this recipe!

Ingredients (makes enough for an 8x8" baking pan):

Mint layer:

- 2 avocados
- 1/2 cup xylitol
- 3/4 cup melted coconut oil

- 1/8 tsp stevia
- 4 cups shredded coconut
- 1/4 tsp peppermint extract
- 1/4 tsp salt
- 3/4 tsp vanilla extract

Chocolate layer:

- 1/2 cup melted coconut oil
- 1/4 cup xylitol
- 1/2 cup cocoa powder
- 1/2 tsp vanilla
- 1/8 tsp salt

Method:

1. Line the baking pan with baking paper or BPA-free cling film.
2. Place all the mint layer ingredients in a high-speed blender. Blend until completely smooth.
3. Spread mixture evenly into the pan and put in the freezer.
4. In a small saucepan, melt coconut oil over low heat and add the xylitol sweetener.
5. Remove from the heat, then add the cacao powder, vanilla and salt. Whisk together until smooth.
6. Pour the chocolate mixture over the chilled mint layer and freeze until the chocolate layer is set - around an hour.

7. Using a warmed knife, cut into bars.
8. Store in an airtight container in the fridge.

Handy Tips

For thinner bars, just go for a bigger baking pan. You can also store these bars in the freezer so they last longer.

BERRY CRUMBLE

My go-to dessert when I need something warm and comforting like a hug. You can make the fruit compote and the crumbly topping separately - the compote can be eaten as a snack with a dollop of peanut butter, while the topping can be made in advance and sprinkled on compote or on smoothie bowls. Enjoy!

Ingredients (serves 4):

For the fruit compote:

- 3 large cooking apples (peeled and chopped)
- 1 cup frozen berries (blackberries, blueberries and raspberries all work)
- 1 cup orange juice
- 1 orange (zest only)
- 1/2 cup dried cranberries
- 1/4 cup chia seeds
- 1 tsp cinnamon

For the crumbly topping:

- 2/3 cup gluten free oats
- 1/3 cup almonds (chopped)
- 1 tbsp coconut oil (melted)
- 2 tbsp xylitol
- 1 tsp vanilla essence

Method:

1. In a bowl, mix together the oats, chopped almonds, coconut oil, xylitol and vanilla essence until well combined.
2. Spread onto a baking tray lined with baking paper, and bake at 400F for 8-12 minutes, until the mixture is golden.
3. Once cooled, this can be stored in an airtight container for up to 2-3 weeks.
4. Place the chopped cooking apples, frozen berries, orange juice and cinnamon in a pan and heat on medium until simmering. Cook for a further 10-15 minutes or until the apple is softened.
5. Stir in the dried cranberries and chia seeds.
6. Keep stirring until the chia seeds have thickened - around 2-3 minutes. Mix in the orange zest.
7. To serve, spoon the fruit compote into a bowl, top with full fat coconut yogurt or oat cream, and a spoonful of crumble topping.

Handy Tips:

- You can swap the almonds in the crumble topping for cashew nuts, or add pumpkin seeds and sunflower seeds instead.
- Instead of cranberries, try sultanas or chopped dried apricots.
- Try different fruits, like peaches and pineapple, for a more tropical dessert.

ALMOND CHIA DESSERT POT

Few things are better than a dessert that actually does your body good. And that's what you get with my almond chia dessert pot. Chia seeds are packed with anti-inflammatory omega-3 and a good amount of gut-friendly fiber. The almond cream makes this little pot taste super indulgent, but it's an indulgence you can feel great about. So healthy, you can even have it for breakfast!

Ingredients (serves 2):

- 1 to 1.5 cup almond cream
- 1/4 cup chia seeds
- 1 tbsp maple syrup or rice syrup (alternatively you can use inulin syrup)
- 1/2 vanilla pod (scraped)

Method:

1. In a bowl, whisk together the chia seeds, almond cream, maple syrup (or sweetener of choice) and vanilla.
2. Leave for ten minutes to thicken, then whisk again until the mix is even. If you find the mixture too thick, or if it is gloopy, add a 1/2 cup more almond cream. Mix well.

3. Cover and refrigerate for at least 2 hours to allow to set.
4. Layer it with fresh berries, top with home-made granola, or enjoy on its own.

Handy Tips:

- Use oat cream or coconut milk instead of almond cream.
- Use 1/2 tsp of cinnamon instead of vanilla.
- Add 1 tbsp of raw cacao powder to make it a chocolate pot.

FINAL WORDS

Studies have shown that 7% of adult women are at risk of being affected by PCOS - and maybe even more. One of the leading factors in PCOS is excess weight, and this problem is brought about by insulin resistance, hormonal imbalance, and inflammation. Even slight weight loss can improve insulin resistance, and therefore improve your PCOS symptoms.

When you lose weight healthily - which means by choosing foods that nourish you, rather than trying to skip meals - you can restore hormone balance, improve insulin sensitivity, and generally enjoy a better quality of life.

In this section, I want to share some weight loss tips. Finding what works for you is the best way to make long-term change. So, take a look at these suggestions and see how you can begin to put them into practice in your own life.

Reduce your carb intake

As we discussed in earlier chapters, carbohydrates impact on your insulin levels, and this in turn impacts on your hormone levels and drives PCOS. According to health experts, close to 70% of women with PCOS are also insulin resistant. This doesn't just trigger weight gain, but also a higher chance of developing diabetes and heart disease.

Since insulin is necessary for managing blood sugar and energy in the body, having the right balance is essential for maintaining a healthy weight. Remember that insulin tells the body to store excess glucose as fat, which means if your body has to pump out lots of insulin in response to high amounts of carbs, you gain body fat. This is the case for anyone, even without PCOS.

Avoid refined carbohydrates completely, and instead focus on getting a small amount of complex carbs, while filling up on plant protein and healthy fats. A low-carb, high protein diet can reset your insulin production - causing the pancreas to produce less insulin, and in turn helping you lose weight and rebalance your hormones.

Key takeaway:

A low-carb, high protein diet helps to reduce the level of insulin in women living with PCOS. This makes weight loss much easier.

Get plenty of fiber

Fiber is essential to keep you feeling full for longer. This means you feel less hungry, and are less likely to snack in between meals. Fiber is also important for PCOS because it slows down the release of sugar in the blood, leading to better insulin management. And finally, it also feeds the good bacteria in your gut - an important part of staying healthy.

Make sure you get plenty of fiber by piling your plate high with vegetables, berries, beans, nuts, seeds and a small amount of whole grains.

Key takeaway:

Switching to a fiber-rich diet can help manage insulin resistance, shed excess weight, and reduce body fat, which in turn helps to manage the symptoms of PCOS.

Get enough protein

Protein is the most filling nutrient, and will help keep your blood sugar levels stable. Foods that help you feel full after a meal will be vital to weight loss, and high-protein foods will do exactly that. You'll be better able to manage your hunger.

If you are worried about the amount of protein in your meals, particularly as you transition to a more plant-based diet, let me put your mind at rest. There is adequate protein in beans, legumes, and certain seeds - plenty for you to get what you need.

Meat is considered a complete protein because it contains all essential amino acids. The good news is that you can find these essential amino acids in buckwheat, quinoa, soy and hemp seeds.

Key takeaway:

Eating plenty of protein will help you feel more satisfied after a meal, which will help you to lose weight.

Add some healthy fats to your diet

Healthy fats also keep you full after meals, which will help you shed excess weight. Many people shy away from fat because of the added calories. But the truth is that healthy fats, like the ones found in olive oil, coconut oil, nuts and seeds, help keep you full for longer and reduce cravings. This means you'll be less likely to over eat or snack during the day, which is one of the best ways to cut down on excess calories and start losing weight.

You might be surprised to know that a diet that includes the right amount of healthy fats is more likely to result in a leaner body mass compared to a low-fat diet (that's because low-fat diets tend to be high in sugar!).

Good examples of healthy fats include nuts and seeds, nut butters (cashew, walnut, almond, etc.), avocado, olive oil, and coconut (flour, butter, oil). Add these in your daily diet with a good amount of protein, and you'll notice a total change in your appetite, and your weight.

Key takeaway:

A diet that includes healthy fats is beneficial to PCOS patients, as it reduces hunger and improves energy, which leads to weight loss.

Eat fermented foods

Did you know that healthy gut bacteria can help with weight loss? One of the reasons for this is that a healthy gut metabolizes food better - that means you absorb more nutrients, which in turn translates to better appetite management. Most health experts agree that women with PCOS have fewer gut bacteria than women without the condition - so it is a good idea to add some back in by eating foods that improve your gut flora.

Fermented foods contain probiotics - this means they contain live bacteria that can help repopulate your gut with friendly organisms.

Examples of fermented foods include organic yogurt, kefir, kimchi (fermented cabbage with ginger and chili), sauerkraut (fermented cabbage), pickles (fermented vegetables), kombucha (fermented tea) and miso (fermented rice paste). Another option is to take a good quality probiotic supplement.

Key takeaway:

Women with PCOS are more likely to have poor gut bacteria compared to their healthy counterparts. Probiotic foods or probiotic supplements will help repopulate gut bacteria, improve nutrient absorption, and aid weight loss.

Eat mindfully

It isn't uncommon for women with PCOS to have tried many different diets. Not only can this be frustrating, but it can open the door the disordered eating. Many of us have learned to eat based on our emotions, or boredom, or to numb our feelings. The result: disrupted appetite, cravings, and weight gain.

What's the antidote to this? Mindful eating. This practice connects you to the act of eating in a way you've probably been missing. When was the last time you were fully present with your meal, and took the time to really savor every mouthful?

When you eat mindfully, you gain a deeper awareness of what your body actually needs. You'll be able to feel when you're full, which means you'll be better able to manage your appetite, and manage your weight. This should not come as a shock since it makes sense that the more attention you pay to what and when you eat, the better you will eat.

Key takeaway:

Mindful eating is the practice of really connecting with your food. Turn off the TV, put away your phone, and focus on every mouthful. You'll find that disordered eating patterns begin to fall away. You'll be conscious of the times when your hunger is motivated by emotions, and find new ways to nourish yourself without binge eating.

Reduce your intake of processed food and added sugar

We don't need to go into this in detail again. After all, we know that processed foods are packed full of sugar - which cause insulin resistance and weight gain. They're also lacking in good quality nutrients. This is why processed foods are also called empty calories: they provide you with calories, often too many, without bringing your body any benefits. Worse, they come with a long list of health risks because they are full of fat and artificial additives, which can increase inflammation and disrupt your hormones.

The result of eating too many processed foods is weight gain, plus a higher risk of chronic disease. Not what you want when you're trying to overcome PCOS symptoms.

It isn't complicated. If you want to rebalance your health, lose weight, improve your hormones and prepare your body for a healthy pregnancy, you must nourish your body - not poison it.

What this means is eating foods that keep your blood sugar levels stable, while delivering real nourishment: whole foods, that have been minimally processed. No added sugars. No refined carbohydrates. What I hope I've shown you with this book is that not eating processed food doesn't mean that you have nothing to eat - you have options, and those options are delicious.

Key takeaway:

Avoid refined carbs and processed foods and replace these with natural, whole, plant-based foods. Forget the cakes, biscuits, crisps, sweets and other junk food, and instead head into your kitchen to make those blueberry cheesecake bites!

Eat foods that reduce inflammation

It's no secret. A diet high in sugar and processed food causes an increase in inflammation. Inflammation is your immune system's way of dealing with problems like infections or injuries - when it is working well, it deals with the issue at hand (for example a cut on your finger) and then goes away. But it can get out of hand if you give your body too many inflammatory foods: like sugar and artificial additives. This type of inflammation, called chronic inflammation, doesn't switch off. Over time, it damages the body and disrupts the way it works. One of the ways that damage manifests is PCOS. But chronic inflammation is also believed to be at the root of almost all chronic diseases - like heart disease and cancer.

The key to lowering inflammation is to stop eating processed foods, but also to favor foods that actively help fight inflammation: anti-inflammatory foods.

What are they? You'll be glad to know you don't have to look very far. Vegetables, fruits, herbs and spices have the highest concentration of antioxidants and anti-inflammatory compounds. Omega-3 is also an excellent anti-inflammatory, well worth adding to your diet.

Key takeaway:

Lower your levels of inflammation and help bring your body back into balance by leaving processed foods on the shelf and instead filling your plate with colorful vegetables.

Do not starve yourself

Your body is a well-designed organism. If you don't give it enough calories, it will release certain hormones, like ghrelin, to increase your appetite. That's why low-calorie diets don't really work - after a few days, all you want to do is eat the entire contents of your fridge.

Starving yourself is not the answer. Skipping meals is not the answer. Not only does it create more hunger, and therefore more likelihood that you will overeat, it also creates the perfect conditions for weight gain. If you're not eating, your body will think that it needs to slow down its metabolism in order to preserve energy - you will end up burning fewer calories. And it might also think it needs to make fat stores in response to this time of famine - result: weight gain!

The best way to achieve a healthy weight is not to stop eating, but rather to change what you're eating. Fill up on vegetables, high protein foods and healthy fats, and you won't need to starve yourself: your weight will naturally normalize. And, with this type of diet, your hormones will also return to balance.

Key takeaway:

Chronic calorie restriction will slow down metabolism and cause weight gain. Don't try to eat less, focus on eating differently instead. Swap the processed foods for whole foods and you'll find your weight drops naturally.

Exercise

We all know that to lose weight, we must exercise. This is even more important when you have PCOS. Exercise helps to improve insulin sensitivity, which in turn may help your body to shed excess body fat. What's more, working out boosts your levels of serotonin, helping you to feel good and reducing depression, one of the symptoms of PCOS.

Whether you join a gym, join a walking group, or simply start small by working out at home, it is imperative that you begin moving your body more. Make time for regular exercise and you will soon notice a difference in your waist and your energy levels.

Key takeaway:

Whatever workout you do, focus on moving your body more every day. Cardio and weight training are helpful when it comes to losing excess body fat and reducing insulin resistance in women with PCOS.

Sleep well and enough

We don't really think of sleep as a weight-loss aid, but it is.

If you don't sleep enough, your body produces excess ghrelin and cortisol, both hormones that stimulate your appetite. That's why when you feel tired, you might also feel an urge to eat. Which explains why people who sleep less than 5 hours a night are more likely to be obese. And why those who sleep less than 6 hours a night have more belly fat than those who sleep between 6 and 8 hours.

On the other hand, proper sleep helps you to manage your weight and improve your health. For every extra hour of sleep, you are giving your body more time in the "rest and digest" mode, where your body can repair and renew itself. And when you wake from a proper night's sleep, you feel energized. You won't need to overeat to boost your energy levels - you'll already have it. More energy to do what you love, to cook, to work out, and to spend time with loved ones.

Key takeaway:

Lack of sleep can cause overeating, excess belly fat, and obesity... and that's without mentioning how irritable you feel when you don't get enough sleep. Making sure you get at least 7 hours a night will help you to improve your energy levels, normalize your appetite, and lose weight. Yes, sleep can do all that. Time to get to bed a little earlier!

Manage your stress

Weight gain is caused by more than just excess calories. Stress can do it too. When you're stressed, your body produces cortisol. High levels of cortisol simulate your appetite, but also lead to higher levels of belly fat. What's more, cortisol increases levels of inflammation, which in turn can exacerbate PCOS. And when you're dealing with PCOS symptoms, it's easy to get stressed... you can see how the cycle can loop, endlessly.

The more you can manage your stress, the less cortisol will be pumping through your body, and this will lower inflammation, help normalize your appetite, and help you lose weight.

How? There are many modalities. The trick is to give yourself a few seconds between a situation and your reaction to it. Yoga, guided meditations, and nature walks can all help to slow you down and help you deal with stressful situations in a calmer way.

Key takeaway:

Chronic stress causes a spike in cortisol, which in turn can increase your appetite and your body fat.

Mindful stress reduction techniques can lower levels of cortisol, and help you manage your weight... and your mood.

Consider taking supplements

Excess hunger can sometimes be due to lacking certain nutrients. That's why it is a good idea to take a high-quality multivitamin, to top up your levels of vitamins and minerals.

Omega-3 is difficult to get in decent amounts from your diet alone, so taking a vegan omega-3 supplement can help - what's more, omega-3 is a powerful anti-inflammatory and has shown promise in helping alleviate depression. Well worth adding to your day!

When choosing supplements, go for reliable brands and check the label to make sure there are not artificial fillers or colors.

Key takeaway:

Top up your nutrient intake with a good quality multivitamin and start lowering your inflammation today with a vegan omega-3 supplement.

***

It has been a privilege to share my journey with you. Thank you again for taking this book into your home. I also hope that you enjoyed my first book, which I found rather therapeutic to write! My goal with these books has been to engage with a much wider audience than my circle of friends and to transform the lives of as many people as possible.

I have discussed the extent to which a full health transformation is possible. The number of PCOS sufferers now able to conceive is inspiring. You may worry about how to incorporate some of the changes mentioned in this book and The PCOS Fix, but you can do anything you set your mind to. Start small, and build from there - you will soon experience the benefits of a healthier lifestyle.

But I also know how hard it can be to overcome years of conditioning and habit. When I first started to put these dietary changes into action, it was chaos in our house for weeks. Thankfully, I have a very patient and understanding husband! At the time, there weren't many cookbooks dedicated to PCOS-friendly recipes. I took great comfort in engaging with the online PCOS community and sharing our kitchen disasters and dining out horror stories! The laughter definitely helped, so I would encourage you to find your community of women that you can share this journey with. I promise they are out there!

In the next section, you'll find my 30-Day PCOS Boot Camp program. It's a week by week program that will take you through the changes you can make to begin showing PCOS the door. Read through it and start putting the advice into practice. Don't worry if you have to adapt it slightly to fit in with your schedule - that is completely okay. What matters is that every day you take a small step towards your goals. Small changes add up to huge transformation.

30-DAY PCOS BOOT CAMP

You have now read two books on how to change your life and overcome PCOS for good. Sometimes, when we first learn about new methods and advice, we can find it hard to know how to put it into practice in our day to day. For that reason, I created this intensive 30-Day PCOS Boot Camp.

There is no point trying to change everything at once - that won't create lasting change. What's more, new habits last longer if you can keep them up for at least 30 days. So, to that end, I have broken down these 30 days into 4 weekly chunks with a bonus 2 days at the end, which should represent the new way to live your life going forward. By the time you get to these last two days of the program, you will notice huge differences in your overall health: your weight will have dropped, you will be less hungry, and sugar, processed food and other unhealthy options will no longer have a hold on you.

This 30-Day Boot Camp includes ideas for meal prep, eating out, food swaps, weekly shopping, as well as caffeine, dairy and gluten consumption. This isn't a strict protocol. Instead, it's about removing the unhealthy foods from your daily diet, and replacing them with delicious foods that support your health, help you lose weight, and tackle PCOS symptoms.

Good luck - and here's to transforming your health, one day at a time.

WEEK ONE

Preparation

Welcome to Week One!

You have made the commitment to get started - congratulations!

Right now, you are probably filled with fear looking at your kitchen cupboards and wondering what you are going to eat! First things first: throw out or give away any food that is not going to make it into your new diet. I'm talking candy, ready meals, chocolate, sweet treats, popcorn, soda - if you have it in your cupboards or your fridge, you are more likely to eat it. And honestly, you really don't want any temptation this week, so try and get your cupboards as bare as possible so you can begin filling them with nourishing alternatives.

When shopping this week, you will need to stock up on new cooking oils. Both olive oil and coconut oil will be the oils of choice. I also suggest you begin to stock up on different spices and herbs, because these are the secret ingredients that will make vegetables taste amazing - you need less salt and sugar when you pack your meals with natural flavor.

This is also the perfect time to make your own trail mix and keep a bag of it handy, as you might find you get hungry and want to snack at various stages of the day. Homemade trail mix can be kept in an airtight container. Use the granola recipe in Chapter 3 as a base, and swap the oats for more seeds.

Invest in a nice, sturdy journal - something that you will be able to write in as you progress on this journey. Use it to note down what you eat and how it makes you feel - this will help you identify emotional triggers to eating, as well as any food sensitivities. Get into the habit of journaling at least once a day. This is a meditative practice that will reconnect you to yourself and help you monitor your progress as you begin to free yourself from PCOS symptoms.

Substitutes and alternatives

For the first week, we really are jumping into the deep end and ticking the biggest culprit off the list first: sugar (and that includes alcohol).

You'll want to be mentally prepared for this, because it could be a rough couple of days as your body will be craving what it has been used to for so long. To that ends, substitutes will help you to transition.

Here are some handy swaps to get you started:

- Swap sugary breakfast cereal with home-made granola (you can have this with sugar-free organic yogurt or vegan milk, and with fruit).
- Swap fizzy drinks for sparkling water with a squeeze of lemon.
- Swap alcohol for mocktails (check out the virgin margarita recipe in Chapter 7).
- Swap candy bars for very dark chocolate (go for varieties that are at least 85% cacao).
- Swap sweet pastries or cakes for blueberry cheesecake, grasshopper bars, or lemon bombs (see Chapter 7 for recipes).

Exercise tips for the week

This week, let's start off gently and just focus on cardio with a few easy-to-pick-up strength exercises thrown in.

Waking up slightly earlier and going for a walk is a great way to kick-start your day, get your blood pumping, and ensure that your metabolism is switched on. Try to finish your walk with a few lunges and always remember to stretch! If you don't have time in the morning, make a point of taking a lunchtime walk instead.

Do a few resistance exercises before you go to bed. Lunges, squats, and sit ups are good options. If you find it too easy, you can fill up two bottles of water and hold them while you exercise. Aim for three sets of 10 to 15 repetitions. The great thing about this is it doesn't take forever, and you don't have to leave your home to engage your muscles. If you find resistance exercise too stimulating before bedtime, try a quick yoga flow instead. YouTube has plenty of videos you can follow.

Shopping tips for the week

Make sure that you have the equipment you need to cook your meals: you'll need a blender, steamer, and slow cooker. You will also want some BPA-free, glass or ceramic storage containers for leftovers and lunches. Many of the meals you will make over the next few weeks can be made in advance, portioned and frozen or kept in the fridge, depending on how quickly you plan to eat them. Lasagna, pasta sauces, chili and soups can all be made in bulk and then divided into portions for later.

Food-wise for this week, I'd like you to really focus on vegetables. Experiment with them. Buy vegetables you've never tried before and cook them. This will help you figure out which ones you love and which ones you don't. At lunch and dinner, make sure that at over half your plate is full of vegetables. Add a handful of kale to your smoothies, dip some raw carrot sticks in hummus as a snack, pile your plate high with salad and drizzle it all in a delicious creamy dressing. However you do it, just make sure you are filling up on veggies.

It's also a good idea to bulk buy some nuts and seeds, gluten-free whole grains, and beans or legumes, so you can begin to restock your empty cupboards with the right ingredients to create tasty, healthy meals.

Watch out for...

...that sugar crash! It might be challenging - especially if you're used to eating it every day. But if anything, it's a sign that you need to quit your reliance on the white stuff. Make sure you always have an alternative to hand. If you feel faint, or irritable, or hungry, have an apple with some peanut butter, or a handful of home-made granola with some fruit. Avoid the candy. Trust me, after a few days, you won't want to go back to that sugar rollercoaster.

Meal plan - Week 1

Begin planning ahead - look at the recipes in this book and decide the meals you'd like to make for lunches and dinner, then schedule some time for batch cooking. Knowing what you will eat ahead of time will stop you from having to make food choices when you're hungry. Make sure you buy everything you need for your meals this week, including enough ingredients to make healthy snacks.

Breakfast will be home-made granola with a green smoothie; lunch will be a protein, complex carbs and some veggies (think Power Bowl), and your evening meal will a portion of protein with a small amount of carbs and a substantial amount of veggies. You can snack on trail mix, nuts, seeds, or fresh berries.

Check out Chapter 5 for the green smoothie recipe. You can adapt this to suit your tastes - for example by adding different vegetables like zucchini or cucumber.

You can still have meat this week, but begin thinking about plant-based options for your power bowls. You can also have some pasta, we are not going gluten-free until Week 3. That said, if you want to fast-track your progress, I recommend switching to gluten-free alternatives, for example brown rice pasta or buckwheat pasta.

Make evening meals as stress-free as possible. Pick one or two recipes from Chapter 6, and cook extra portions so you have leftovers ready for the rest of the week. If you are eating your evening meal late at night, increase the amount of vegetables and protein and keep your carbs to a minimum. Even complex carbs, like squash or lentils, can be a bit heavy on the stomach right before bed. Aim to have your evening meal at least three hours before going to bed - this way, digestion won't disrupt your sleep.

WEEK TWO

Preparation

Well done on completing Week One! Week Two will be much the same, but this time you already know what you're doing, and you've got the basics in the kitchen, ready to go.

The only small changes you will want to make to your shopping list this week might be to try and pick up a few more cooking substitutes like dairy alternatives, for example almond milk, to help you transition away from animal protein and towards healthier plant protein.

By now, you should know your key vegetables - these are the ones you love the taste of. It makes sense to stock up on these vegetables and include them in your meals. The more vegetables, the better. This week, try out some different herbal teas. Next week, we will remove caffeine, so you will need some alternatives at the ready.

Here is the real preparation for this week: I would like you to start incorporating some mindfulness and meditation practices into your morning. You can prepare for this by deciding when you have time for meditation - you can use a guide like Waking Up or

Headspace to help you along. You will now have a week of journaling under your belt and you might feel a little bit more in control of your mornings. Hopefully, you are also seeing the benefits of including gentle movement into your day. Keep going, don't drop any of these new habits, and try to set aside 10 minutes or so per day to center yourself, and feel connected to your purpose in healing your body.

Another thing to think about this week is to reduce your feeding window to 12 hours maximum. For example, eating between 7am and 7pm or 8am and 8pm, and only having water or herbal tea outside these windows. This will help your digestion, and give your body time in a fasted state, where it can repair and rejuvenate itself.

Substitutes and alternatives

This is the week we really start to tackle dairy. So the key foods we are going to substitute this week are milk and cheese.

You now have many options for vegan cheese - you'll have to try different brands to find one that works for you! As for milk, there are plenty of tasty alternatives that you can use in coffee, tea, breakfast cereal, and any baking. Try coconut milk, almond milk, oat milk, hemp milk and soy milk. You might want different ones for different things. For example, oat milk works well in coffee, while almond milk is a good addition to granola.

Obviously, that caramel latte from Starbucks is no longer part of your life, since we gave up sugar last week - however that doesn't mean you can't enjoy an oat latte or coconut latte - just have the coffee without the syrup. Why not try sprinkling a little cinnamon in there instead? Make the most of it, because next week we'll be cutting out the caffeine!

Exercise tips for the week

It's time to step it up slightly. This week, I would like you to incorporate a yoga practice. Not as a substitute for your daily walk and exercise, but as an addition.

To start, try some of the short yoga workouts you can find on YouTube and get yourself used to the positions in the comfort of your own home. Practice in front of a mirror, so you can check your alignment. Pick classes or videos that are in line with your current ability - if you've never tried yoga before, trying to follow a complicated asana flow will only be frustrating. Yin yoga is a good place to start, since it is slow and easier to follow.

After this week, I'm going to encourage you to pick up a regular gym routine and maybe even get a personal trainer, so make the most of this time to get comfortable with your commitment to your fitness. Treat yourself to some new yoga pants, a nice bright mat, and some gym sneakers.

Shopping tips for the week

Only buy the fruits and foods you enjoy. As you start to cut more out of your diet, like dairy, you will crave some pleasure in your diet. Don't be scared to increase your portion size this week if you feel hungry - your body is getting used to new habits and might be craving more. If you increase portion sizes, focus on vegetables and protein instead of carbohydrates. The most important thing is that you do not revert back to dairy or sugar, and that you start reducing your dependency on carbs. You might be surprised at just how much good food you can eat, while still losing weight.

Watch out for...

...the changes that avoiding dairy will make to your life! You might start to notice your sinuses feel clearer, your nose stops running, and you no longer cough or feel congested. You will also start to notice your face is less puffy, the bags under your eyes are reduced, and you feel more energetic.

Meal plan

Last week, we enjoyed a home-made granola for breakfast as a way to transition from the high sugar alternatives that we were eating previously. This week, let's make breakfast lighter by having just the green smoothie. If you find this is too little, then go with a high-protein low-carb option, for example scrambled tofu or hard-boiled eggs on wilted spinach.

WEEK THREE

Preparation

As the weeks progress, your food preparation should be getting easier and you should now be ahead of the game! For this week your preparation will center more on mental changes rather than tangible dietary changes.

This is the week that we will be removing caffeine from our diets. If there is any one substance this is habit-forming and impacts the structure of our day, it is coffee. Replacing it, therefore, is more of a mental exercise than a physical one, so this is the week where you want to cement your journaling habits, meditation, and mindfulness practices.

When you feel yourself craving that cup of coffee, come back to the present moment. Turn your attention to why you're making these changes in the first place. The more you master this, the more confidence you will gain within yourself, and the easier it will be to stick with your new habits long term.

Substitutes and alternatives

There are many things you can substitute coffee for. Organic decaffeinated coffee is one - in fact this is a great way to give yourself the flavor of coffee without the cortisol spike. There is no point trying to substitute every cup of coffee for a cup of herbal tea - it just isn't going to work, they are too dissimilar.

So, try to keep the timings of your drinks the same, but instead of having caffeine, have a caffeine-free alternative (decaf coffee or decaf tea, with a splash of coconut milk or oat milk, for example). This will trick your brain into believing that you've satisfied your craving.

Another substitute that I haven't really touched on yet is not dietary, but content-related. If you've read The PCOS Fix, you will know about the benefits of doing a digital detox. By reducing the amount of time you spend on your phone or in front of a screen, you reduce the amount of stress in your life and give yourself better sleep as well.

So why not swap some of your screen time for a hobby or other activity? It could be something social like a walk with the girls, or something creative like painting or pottery. Or maybe you've got a pile of books you've been meaning to read but haven't ever got around to. Try something different, at least one night a week. Learning new things builds new neural connections in our brains, and this can help you stick to healthy habits.

Exercise tips for the week

This leads in nicely to my exercise tips for the week. You've been walking, doing some home workouts, doing a little yoga… now it's time to add something different. It's time to get back to the gym. Most gyms offer a free personal training session when you join - make the most of this offer. Tell the trainer the work you've been doing so far, and your goals. Ask them to show you the best resistance exercises and cardio to build your fitness and reduce body fat.

Shopping tips for the week

You should already have well-stocked cupboards by this point and all of your dairy and sugar should now be gone, with healthy vegan alternatives in their place. Now it's time to get a bit more adventurous. As we move towards more plant-based dishes, start looking for healthy meat alternatives to add to your diet.

You could also invest in some new home workout equipment this week, in the form of resistance bands, weights, or kettlebells. This is a good idea because there are times when you really don't want to hit the gym - having some equipment at home means you will still be able to exercise and work those muscles.

Watch out for...

...caffeine headaches! Depending how much coffee you usually drink, you might experience headaches as you go caffeine-free. If you do, reduce your intake gradually, for example, start with having just one coffee a day for a few days, before transitioning to no coffee. These headaches are simply your body reacting to the fact it isn't getting something that it's used to. Giving coffee up for a little while will help your body to readjust and return to normal. The positive of this is that next time you have coffee, you'll be able to feel the full effect.

Meal plan

By now, your breakfast routine is pretty much sorted, but let's mix it up a bit. Increase your consumption of healthy proteins, like eggs and avocados, at breakfast. Poached eggs with smashed avocado make a tasty and filling breakfast. Or you can opt for a healthy omelet, with peppers, mushrooms and chili flakes, to really bring up the heat.

We really want to reduce some of our meat dishes this week. So, for your power bowls, make sure you're including plant protein (tofu, beans, bean burgers) or eggs instead of meat or poultry. Use different bases for your salads to keep things interesting, for example using spinach or romaine lettuce instead of kale, swapping the brown rice for quinoa, or adding some sweet complex carbs like sweet potato or pumpkin, and making sure there's some raw veggies in there as well, for texture (tomatoes, cucumber, celery, radish, etc.). Always add a homemade dressing - dressings make veggies irresistible.

For evening meals, you should now have transitioned to having at least two or three meat-free days per week. Try to increase this to three or four. Include some of the healthy plant-based options and season them in the same way you would a beef burger or steak. Make low-carb burgers by using lettuce leaves instead of buns. Why not try cooking outdoors on a BBQ, and make kebabs using soy-based meats, peppers, corn, mushrooms... This week is about trying out some new cooking styles and experimenting with different meat-free options. The more you cook with plants, the easier it will be. You'll soon see that it is just as tasty, if not tastier, than traditional meat-centric meals.

WEEK FOUR

Preparation

You can take your foot slightly off the gas this week, as most of the hard work has been done. You will be an expert at meal prep by now and your metabolism will have adjusted to your new healthy routine. In Week Four, focus on the timing of your meals. Reduce your eating window to about 10 hours and aim to get your walk, workout, and some meditation time in the morning before having your smoothie. How this looks in practice is that you might have your breakfast at around 8 or 9am, and have dinner by 6 or 7pm. Play around with timings to find what works for you.

Substitutes and alternatives

This week, experiment with low-carb versions of your usual grains. For example, did you know that you can make rice from cauliflower or broccoli? By simply pulsing the florets in a food processor, you can break down the vegetables into rice-sized pieces, and then use that as a replacement for grains. You can have it raw for a crunchy texture, or lightly fry it in coconut oil with some spices or herbs.

Try to minimize your intake of grains this week. Include root vegetables like beetroot, sweet potato, pumpkin, and carrots instead. These provide some complex carbs alongside vitamins and minerals. Plus, they are delicious roasted and make a flavorful alternative to white potatoes.

Now is also the time to get a bit more experimental with some of the vegetables that you might have avoided earlier in the program. Your taste buds have now changed, and can appreciate different flavors. Hopefully, you took my advice and invested in a good steamer, so that you can layer and cook different vegetables at the same time. Pile them high on your plate, drizzle them in dressing or simply sprinkle some toasted seeds on top and enjoy!

Exercise tips for the week

You now have a regular workout routine, and you've brought in a weekly activity to ensure you don't get bored. This week, start thinking about your long-term fitness goals. Maybe you could sign up for a half marathon, or even a marathon! Push yourself towards a goal that you may think is unachievable right now. Four weeks ago, this life would have seemed unachievable, so you know you can do it if you put your mind to it!

Shopping tips for the week

Head to your local farmer's market - this is where you'll find the most organic vegetables, as well as varieties that aren't usually in supermarkets. Pick out three or four and experiment with them. Don't be afraid to ask for recipe inspiration.

Buy one or two spice mixes that you've not tried before. This will give you even more options when you come to cook your meals, and will make your plant-based dishes even more interesting.

This is the week you will venture out and try your new lifestyle in a restaurant setting. So take a moment to research healthy restaurants near you, or browse the menu of your favorite place and use your skills to work out which dish is healthy, or how some of their dishes could be made healthier. It might be tempting to never eat out again, but that's not sustainable - there are plenty of options out there so don't be afraid. You can have a healthy lifestyle and still enjoy yourself - remember the 80/20 rule.

Watch out for...

...hitting that plateau! At this stage, you might feel like you have hit a plateau when it comes to your weight loss or your fitness. The drastic changes you experienced in the first few weeks can't last forever, but you must not let this discourage you or dissuade you from keeping up with your new habits.

Your emotions, your body, and your mental health should all be seeing significant improvements from all the hard work you have put in over the last few weeks. And, if you need reminding of how far you've come, read back through your journal from when you started this plan. You should be really proud of yourself and all that you have achieved!

Meal plan

This week, you should continue to focus on eating plenty of vegetables, plenty of plant-protein, and some healthy fats. When you eat out, go for low-carb options and think about the hidden ingredients (ask the waiter about salad dressings or sauces, and see if they can be swapped or served on the side).

Breakfast should be as light as possible, just have a smoothie. If you're eating later to stick with a shorter eating window, you can simply take it to work and have it as a mid or late morning snack.

Get a bit creative with your lunchtime power bowls. Maybe swap the brown rice for cauliflower rice, or experiment with a new dressing. Why not try gluten-free pasta made from buckwheat? Take your favorite combinations and switch them up a bit. Keep it varied and interesting.

For dinner, test yourself by going out and making some healthy choices. Choose vegetarian or vegan restaurants and use their menus to inspire your own home cooking. Remember to choose the low-carb options and don't be afraid to ask the waiter for swaps (for example steamed vegetables instead of fries). After all your hard work the last three weeks, you may find that you're not craving the same foods you used to. Be careful to not take your foot off the gas so much that you end up back in your old habits - this is the week to get a feel for how your healthy eating regime will last in the long term, instead of being a one-month wonder!

Day 29 and 30

Congratulations - you made it! Your diet is low-carb, you've reconnected with the joy of vegetables, you're incorporating movement and meditation into every day - you are now living your perfect life! The end of the month is a great time to just look back over what you have achieved and see the differences that all these changes made in your life. Take a moment to pat yourself on the back for getting here. Sit down and plan ahead - how will you keep up these healthy habits next month?

By now, you will have a regular routine. Below, I've outlined what mine looks like. Don't worry if the timings don't completely match up - after all, we live diverse lives with diverse schedules!

- 6.30am - wake up.
- Go for a walk; do some yoga.
- Journal, meditate, get ready for the day.
- 11am - green smoothie.
- 2pm - power bowl lunch - a good mix of protein, veg, and small amount of complex carbs.
- Healthy snack if needed.
- 7pm - evening meal - high protein, lots of veggies.
- Workout / social activity, rest and relaxation.
- 9pm - digital detox - zero screen time, herbal tea.
- 10pm - sleep.

Just imagine how great you will feel when you have taken control of your diet and your daily schedule in this way. You will see the difference in the mirror and on the scales; your hormones and your emotions will be balanced. Your PCOS symptoms will be a thing of the past. It is worth the hard work and I wish you the very best of luck in coming out the other side stronger, healthier, and happier.

Don't delay - start making changes today.

Printed in Great Britain
by Amazon